Modernising Cancer Services

Edited by
Mark R Baker

Foreword by
Professor Mike Richards
National Cancer Director

Radcliffe Medical Press

Radcliffe Medical Press Ltd
18 Marcham Road
Abingdon
Oxon OX14 1AA
United Kingdom

www.radcliffe-oxford.com
The Radcliffe Medical Press electronic catalogue and online ordering facility.
Direct sales to anywhere in the world.

British Library Cataloguing in Publication Data

A catalogue record for this book is available from the British Library.

ISBN 1 85775 459 X

Typeset by Aarontype Ltd, Easton, Bristol
Printed and bound TJ International Ltd, Padstow, Cornwall

Contents

Foreword

Cancer is a major health problem in the UK. At least one in three people will be diagnosed with cancer during their lifetime and one in four die from it. Sadly, cancer services in this country have been under-funded for decades. As a result we have too few trained staff and inadequate facilities. This under-investment has led to unacceptably long waiting times for diagnosis and treatment. Most importantly, survival rates for patients in the UK have, in the past, been well below the European average. In addition, there are inequalities within the UK in relation to who gets cancer and who dies from cancer – with deprived people faring worse.

Modernising Cancer Services charts the progress that has been made following the publication of the Calman–Hine Report in 1995 and the NHS Cancer Plan in 2000. The authors – commissioners, providers, managers, researchers and a recipient of cancer care – are recognised experts who have been at the forefront of cancer services in this country. They give valuable insights into the improvements which have been made and the challenges which lie ahead. *Modernising Cancer Services* will, I believe, be of interest to the huge numbers of staff and patients who are committed to bringing the quality of cancer care in this country up to the level of the best in Europe.

Professor Mike Richards CBE
National Cancer Director
April 2002

Preface

Evidence that people with cancer in the UK receive less specialist care and experience poorer outcomes than in many other countries has been accumulating now for several years. Although not all of this evidence stands up to critical enquiry, there is certainly a case to answer in terms of the timeliness, completeness and expertise of some cancer treatment in this country. As one-third of people will experience cancer at some time in their lives, the optimal management of cancer is a major public health and clinical management issue.

Improving the care of people with cancer in order to enhance their experience of the services and to secure better outcomes is a leading clinical priority of the UK Government. Close co-ordination of public health goals (*Saving Lives: Our Healthier Nation*), NHS developments (the *NHS Cancer Plan*) and improved organisation and content of clinical services (*Improving Outcomes Guidance*), have provided a coherent framework for addressing the shortfall in services and survival.

In this book, a wide range of specialists have contributed to a comprehensive overview of the challenges facing cancer services in the UK and the responses now being planned and/or implemented. The general approach is optimistic because, whatever practical difficulties are inherent in today's NHS, it is clear that the Government, people and health professionals of this country have a common goal; better care and better outcomes for people with cancer.

Mark R Baker
April 2002

List of contributors

Professor Mark R Baker
Director and Lead Clinician
Yorkshire Cancer Network

Mitzi Blennerhassett
Patient

May Bullen
Lead Nurse
Kent Cancer Network

Dr Carol Chu
Consultant Clinical Geneticist
Leeds Teaching Hospitals

Professor David Forman
Director of Research and Information
Northern and Yorkshire Cancer Registry

Dr Anne Garry
Consultant in Palliative Medicine
York District Hospital

Dr Geoff Hall
Senior Lecturer/Honorary Consultant in Medical Oncology
Imperial Cancer Research Fund Clinical Centre
Leeds

Dr Anita Hatfield
Consultant in Public Health Medicine
Calderdale and Kirklees Health Authority

Professor Robert Haward
Director
Northern and Yorkshire Cancer Registry

Dr Rosemary Macdonald
Former Postgraduate Dean
Yorkshire Deanery
University of Leeds

Dr Ian Manifold
Medical Director and Clinical Oncologist
Weston Park Hospital
Sheffield

Dr Michael Peake
Consultant in Respiratory Medicine
Glenfield Hospital
Leicester

Dr Tim Perren
Senior Lecturer/Consultant in Medical Oncology
ICRF Cancer Medicine Research Unit
Leeds Teaching Hospitals

Professor Peter Selby
Director
ICRF Cancer Medicine Research Unit
University of Leeds

Dr Nicholas Summerton
Senior Lecturer in Primary Care
University of Hull

Dr Roger Taylor
Consultant Clinical Oncologist
Leeds Teaching Hospitals

Dr John Wilkinson
Director
Northern and Yorkshire Public Health Observatory

CHAPTER I

Introduction: cancer – a suitable case for treatment

Mark R Baker

Origins of the problem

Under-investment

International comparisons have clearly demonstrated that cancer services in the UK have failed to keep pace with those in other countries across a wide range of measures. There has been widespread under-investment in key facilities used in cancer care, including linear accelerators and chemotherapy for treatment and pathology and imaging services for diagnosis. In particular, the slow roll-out of computerised tomography and magnetic resonance imaging has compared poorly with that in other countries.

Lack of specialisation

The training of surgeons in the UK, both in general surgery and in other surgical subspecialties, has followed a generic course for most of the history of the NHS. Only in recent years have the major subspecialties such as urology and vascular surgery enjoyed separate training programmes and accreditation. Within general surgery, gynaecology and head and neck surgery, the introduction of specialist accreditation for surgical oncology and the separate designation of specialisation in breast, colorectal and upper gastrointestinal cancer surgery has been a recent phenomenon. As a result, most cancer surgery is performed by surgeons carrying a general workload, and true specialisation is uncommon.

Non-surgical oncology

Along with the deficiencies in linear accelerators, there has been a systematic failure to train sufficient numbers of clinical and medical oncologists. The previously mainly academic specialty of medical oncology has developed rapidly during the last decade such that it is now easier to recruit medical oncologists than clinical oncologists. However, their numbers remain small relative to the whole non-surgical oncology establishment, and training programmes have failed to keep pace with the now emerging demand in both specialties. As a consequence, the likelihood of a cancer patient in the UK being seen by a cancer specialist is low compared with that in other countries. In addition, site specialisation in non-surgical oncology has been difficult to organise, with insufficient staff and small teams working out of cancer centres.

Histopathology

A substantial proportion of the work of histopathology departments is cancer related. One calculation (P Quirk, personal communication) suggests that 50% of the workload is directly related to cancer and a further 25% is aimed at excluding cancer. As mentioned above, failed workforce planning arrangements and a lack of specialisation in site specificity has resulted in understaffed departments and fragmented provision of specialist advice.

Resource limitations

The desire of advocates of better cancer services to redress the above deficiencies has been seriously constrained by recurrent financial difficulties, and was further compromised by the mechanisms of the NHS internal market, which rendered difficult additional investment in specialist regional services such as radiotherapy. These problems have subsequently been overcome to some extent by the regional arrangements for commissioning specialist services, although they now appear to be under threat again from the devolution of commissioning to primary care trusts.

Hospital planning

The overall shortage of capital development in the NHS and the genre of developing local services through district general hospitals in small and medium-sized towns has created a highly fragmented, although accessible NHS. With most of the available capital going towards the development of local hospitals, it has rarely been possible to develop centres of excellence for cancer care in which the modalities of treatment (surgery, radiotherapy and chemotherapy) are co-located.

Professional constraints

In addition to lack of specialisation and under-staffing, behaviour patterns in the medical profession have also been an obstacle to progress. In particular, the conflicting effects of private practice and specialisation have compromised the latter and continue to do so. The private sector has paid little heed to the evidence relating to specialisation and outcomes, and the few role models who do exist have often been disbelieved by their peer group. These constraints have applied equally to diagnostic and treatment specialties, and have rarely been challenged by NHS managers.

Information and audit

The most reliable information on cancer incidence and outcomes comes from the cancer registration process which is regionally based and nationwide. However, registries do not normally hold comprehensive information on what treatments are offered or by whom, and there has been relatively little research on the effect of service organisation on cancer outcomes. Although a number of large audits of site-specific cancers have demonstrated powerful relationships between the volume of work done by surgeons (as a proxy for specialisation) or hospitals and better outcomes, no comprehensive database exists.

Patient empowerment

As with other aspects of healthcare in the UK, patients have insufficient information to be able to be fully involved in decisions about their care, or to be aware who should be offering them which treatments. There has been substantial development of self-help groups and lobbying organisations for cancer patients during the last decade or two, but these are focused principally on breast cancer, and self-help groups tend to be dominated by women patients.

Palliative care

The failure of the NHS to handle dying well led to the initiative in palliative care being taken by the voluntary sector. As voluntary giving operates best when it is centred around a building, the model of palliative care that was developed was largely institutional, with the result that a small number of patients received excellent care, but the majority received little palliative care.

Lack of a cancer strategy

Although individual professional groups and medical Royal Colleges produced reports from time to time on the need to increase investment and improve organisation with regard to cancer, these approaches were fragmented, sometimes conflicting and rarely supported in practice. Furthermore, most such reports were watered down in a way which would not upset the majority of professional members. The NHS itself did not have a cancer strategy, and there was no single constituency within the healthcare sector which was empowered to co-ordinate the development of a cancer strategy.

Consequential outcomes

It is hardly surprising, in the context of the above, that outcomes for cancer patients in the UK compare relatively poorly with those in similar countries. Access to specialists, availability of treatments and survival rates are all significantly lower than in many other developed nations. Successive governments have set targets for reducing deaths from cancer, but envisaged that the main tools for doing so would be a reduction in cigarette smoking as well as screening programmes for breast and cervical cancer.[1,2] The role of treatment in achieving cure has generally been underplayed.

Longstanding experience of negative outcomes has tended to generate pessimism within the health professions as well as among the general public with regard to a diagnosis of cancer, and a repetitive cycle of nihilism and negativism has been created. Symptomatic of this has been a lack of urgency, both within primary care and in the hospital sector, in dealing promptly with patients who have symptoms suggestive of cancer. The consequential fear of cancer among members of the public reduces their sensitivity to symptoms and signs, and this can cause further delay in presentation.

The combination of multiple system delays in accessing treatment, inadequate specialist care and overall lack of resources for diagnosis and treatment of cancer contributes significantly to the poor outcomes experienced in this country.

Steps to recovery

The Calman–Hine Report

An expert advisory group on cancer was established by the Chief Medical Officers of England and Wales in 1994. The eponymous Calman–Hine Report[3] was published the following year and described many of the above features. It outlined a framework for the management of cancer patients, including the designation of cancer units and cancer centres, and it also focused strongly on the need to expand the knowledge base and role of primary care and to develop services which were much more patient centred.

As an example of central planning introduced at the height of the NHS internal market, the report had a surprisingly strong impact, and it would be fair to say that nothing in the NHS has been quite the same since. In its White Paper, *The New NHS*,[4] the present Government described the Calman–Hine Report as a National Service Framework for cancer, and regarded it as the model for promoting improvements in other services. Frameworks have subsequently been published for mental health, coronary heart disease and services for older people, and many others are planned. In fact, the Calman–Hine Report is not remotely like a National Service Framework. However, it has been described by its authors as an invitation to write a National Service Framework.

Improving outcomes guidance

The detail of service changes, which we have come to expect in a National Service Framework, was initiated through the commissioning of a series of manuals from the then Clinical Outcomes Group. This work has now been taken over by the National Institute for Clinical Excellence, but the format and purpose of the documents have survived several changes of ownership, and all of them are published under the general heading *Improving Outcomes in Cancer*. The procedure adopted for this work is described in Chapter 7, and the series will not be complete until the end of 2002. The general approach has been evidence based, and recommendations have been informed both by clinical trials and by well-constructed clinical audits.

The first three manuals dealt with the common cancers (breast, lung and colorectal) and principally focused on the team approach to treatment and the organisation of local services. Subsequent volumes dealing with the inter-mediate-frequency cancers (gynaecological, upper gastrointestinal and urologi-cal) have recommended significant service reconfigurations in addition. It is these service shifts, accompanied by major investment and very highly special-ised units, which begin to reach the heart of the problem. There has been signifi-cant if muted opposition to the changes proposed, but the guidance has the confidence of Government and the medical Royal Colleges, and its full implemen-tation is essential if cancer services are to be truly modernised. The introduction of the system of clinical governance places a major responsibility on trust man-agers, as well as the professions, to concentrate on what they do well and often, and to refer less common conditions to specialists in cancer centres. This runs counter to the culture of the NHS internal market and also to the career expecta-tions of many doctors in hospitals, and the transition will not be easy.

The NHS Cancer Plan

The NHS Cancer Plan,[5] which was published in September 2000, remains some-thing of an enigma. It is not really a strategy, but more a series of tactics and targets and a description of drivers for change which are already in the system. In common with its parent publication, the NHS Plan,[6] it focuses on aspects of modernisation such as reducing waiting times in the system and promoting the empowerment and involvement of patients. Major increases in the numbers of staff involved in cancer care are promised, but these merely reflect the impact of the output of existing training programmes in England – except for nursing, where the expansion in staff numbers relies on returners to work or immigra-tion. There is also a modest investment programme in radiotherapy and imaging facilities which provides a degree of catch-up for the deficiencies of the last few years. The most interesting aspects of the Cancer Plan already had a momentum of their own (the adoption of national standards of practice, the Cancer Research Network, the Cancer Information Strategy and the Cancer Services Collabora-tive). The distinctive and enduring feature of the Cancer Plan was the role of cancer networks in implementing change.

The role of cancer networks

In most parts of the country, cancer networks were established in the aftermath of the Calman–Hine Report. The term *cancer network* is used in that report to describe a type of relationship between cancer units and a cancer centre. In some parts of the country the focus was on establishing and developing cancer centres, especially in smaller and more remote hospitals with radiotherapy facilities. In better established centres, the emphasis was on developing secure clinical pathways between units and the centre, and in the most developed areas it incorporated collective commissioning of cancer centre services across an entire network. The more advanced clinical networks had developed agreed protocols for the major cancers and a broadly based set of site-specific and generic clinical groups. Managerially, most cancer networks were semi-virtual organisations run by volunteers with limited administrative support. The NHS Cancer Plan changes all of that.

Cancer networks are deemed to be responsible for implementing the NHS Cancer Plan, although the accountability for doing so remains with the statutory organisations which are members of the network. This little conundrum interests many people but has achieved resolution from none. Network management arrangements and leadership are described in the *Manual of Cancer Services Standards*[7] (see below), and effectively involve the conversion of cancer networks from semi-virtual organisations into real and managed organisations of a significant scale. Subsequent actions by the Cancer Action Team at the Department of Health have continued to focus on networks as the first port of call for various initiatives, including the holding of funds, and for the co-ordination of all of the activities described below.

Manual of Cancer Services Standards

The *Manual of Cancer Services Standards* provides a vehicle for a two-pronged appraisal of cancer services. This manual, which was published in December 2000, contains over 800 standards for hospitals, cancer units/centres and cancer networks which focus on a range of aspects of implementing the NHS Cancer Plan and *Improving Outcomes Guidance*. Cancer centres, networks and units were asked to conduct a self-assessment against these standards during the first few months of 2001, and this was followed by a peer-review-visiting process during the following summer. The gap analysis resulting from these assessments provides the basis for medium-term service improvement plans on both a local and a network-wide basis. The existing standards are based on those piloted in the Trent region several years ago. The current national standards will be further extended in the future to encompass aspects of primary care and palliative care, as well as taking into account subsequent manuals of *Improving Outcomes Guidance*. Experience from those regions in the vanguard of this process suggests that the peer review visits are extremely useful for focusing on the most urgent priorities, and that self-assessment provides a sound basis for medium- to long-term plans to improve services.

National Cancer Research Network

In a recent review of the NHS Research and Development Strategy's priorities, the highest priority in the cancer section was to improve the infrastructure for cancer research in the NHS. The National Cancer Research Network provides that infrastructure and will eventually cover every cancer network in the UK.

Unlike most of the above, the National Cancer Research Network covers the whole of the UK and not just England. The network is intended, among other things, to double the number of patients with cancer who are entered into clinical trials over a three-year period, while also accelerating the generation of knowledge and securing stronger links between the funders of research, those who determine the priorities for research and the operational services. More than £20 million per annum will be spent on resourcing the National Cancer Research Network, which is likely to become a permanent feature of cancer services in this country, although its current funding is only guaranteed for five years.

The resources available for the National Cancer Research Network will be applied equally across the whole country on a formula basis, such that each network will have clinical and administrative leadership and research support staff in its hospitals. A national co-ordinating centre based in Leeds and working with the MRC's clinical trials unit will pull the whole show together and co-ordinate the work of both cancer research networks in the NHS and the national level work on setting priorities and agreeing funding for trials.

Cancer information

Prompt and high-quality clinical information is at the heart of any clinical networking arrangement. One of the fundamental weaknesses of the NHS has been its inability to generate patient-related information which is of value to clinicians. A Cancer Information Strategy was published in the summer of 2000 which envisaged the development of a comprehensive clinical information database that would provide the basis for both current clinical recording and group information at the level of clinician, diagnosis, cancer unit and cancer network. There have been prolonged delays in delivering agreed minimum datasets for individual cancers, although these are now starting to be implemented in some networks. There has been equal chaos in terms of the funding of the Cancer Information Strategy, with the cancer constituency seeking to call on the funds associated with the implementation of the NHS Information Strategy

(Information for Health), while the custodians of these funds regard the Cancer Information Strategy as a matter for those who hold designated funds for the implementation of the NHS Cancer Plan. These games are of course both unhelpful and pointless, but the matter is still unresolved at the time of going to press.

An important and related issue concerns the development and dissemination of information for patients with cancer, and this has received disappointingly little attention. As is too often the case, matters concerning patient empowerment are being progressed most effectively by the voluntary sector and not by the NHS itself. This is sadly symptomatic of NHS managerial and professional attitudes to users of services, and it is up to cancer networks to change this culture by putting the needs of patients at the centre of their strategies, information and service. There is substantial evidence that well-prepared and properly presented information for patients can have a significant impact on the choice of treatment and therefore probably also on compliance. An effect on outcome has not yet been demonstrated, but patient empowerment is a legitimate goal in its own right and does not necessarily have to be 'legitimised' by evidence of a beneficial effect on outcome.

Cancer Services Collaborative

The collaborative genre is based on health improvement science which is evidence based but not research based. In short, a clinical team attempts to improve services by trying out new ideas and responding in a way that is appropriate to their observations. If an idea works, it is implemented, and if an idea is unsuccessful, it is dropped. These principles are being applied to a number of service areas in the NHS, including primary care, orthopaedics and cancer services. The primary objective is to reduce delays in the pathway of care, especially between referral and treatment. Initial experience suggests that major progress can be made in this area without committing significant additional resources to service infrastructure, but the process also exposes bottlenecks and potential conflicts between cancer services and non-cancer services, and challenges the way in which hospital services have been constructed in the UK over many years.

The opportunity exists to make links between the Primary Care Collaborative and the Cancer Services Collaborative, particularly in the time frame prior to referral, to further reduce the delays in the diagnosis and treatment of patients with cancer. Although the Cancer Services Collaborative is essentially designed to improve the process of care, a comprehensively successful approach could well be accompanied by improvements in the outcomes of care both by reducing the stage of cancer at presentation and by sharpening up the whole system of care.

Tensions

The development of the cancer strategy has not been without difficulties, and will doubtless continue to identify barriers to progress during the remaining years of its life. The Calman–Hine Report itself exposed a number of challenges with regard to what constituted a cancer centre, and whether units in remote areas should continue to provide radiotherapy services and on what basis. The riders in the Calman–Hine Report about defining a cancer centre as more than simply a building have encouraged a more liberal interpretation in some areas, including the idea of a cancer centre being a virtual organisation in which elements of highly specialised services may be provided in a number of semi-remote locations. This is not what the authors had in mind, and it may serve to water down the benefits of implementing the new model.

Improving Outcomes Guidance and reconfiguring services

As described elsewhere, an extensive programme of guidance is being produced to help to shape future services for patients with cancer, and to ensure that a high and equal quality of care (the principal aspiration of the Calman–Hine Report) is delivered throughout the country. While the early volumes of guidance, covering the common cancers (breast, lung and colorectal cancer), focused principally on the development of multidisciplinary approaches to managing these cancers in cancer units, the guidance on intermediate-frequency cancers frequently proposes a degree of centralisation and other service reconfiguration. For example, the guidance on gynaecological cancers and gastrointestinal cancers is highly centralising in terms of surgical oncology, and this has stimulated the anticipated opposition from clinicians working in cancer units. The difficulties involved in implementing this guidance include both the creation of specialist service capacity within cancer centres and the persuasion of cancer unit clinicians that such centralisation is necessary and desirable in order to realise the benefits described in the manuals of guidance. Clinicians have highlighted the risks of deskilling clinicians in cancer units, with a potential impact on non-oncology services and especially the handling of emergencies. Although their case is often exaggerated, these concerns are not entirely without foundation, and a means of both realising the benefits of implementing the strategy for cancer and also protecting the quality and viability of general acute services needs to be found. The full implementation of the guidance would undoubtedly pose a challenge to the integrity of acute surgical rotas in these specialties in cancer units, and may call into question the future organisation of general acute services in smaller hospitals.

The focus of the debate over implementing *Improving Outcomes Guidance* for intermediate cancers on the issues of centralisation has distracted attention from the many other elements of service improvement that the guidance promotes. This is particularly true of the development of local diagnostic services and substantial enhancement of non-surgical oncology services.

Workforce capacity

All of the guidance documents encourage the NHS to increase specialisation and subspecialisation in a wide range of specialties and professions, as well as specific increases in specialties which are already in short supply, such as clinical oncology and histopathology. In addition, the establishment of specialist surgical oncology units (e.g. for gynaecological cancers and upper gastrointestinal cancers) creates a new type of surgical post which may be difficult to fill, not least because of the limited opportunities for private practice. Conversely, local opposition to centralisation is to some extent influenced by the potential loss of private practice in oncological fields.

The substantial increases in consultant numbers in a wide range of specialties have been outlined in the NHS Cancer Plan, and these have stretched credibility among members of the medical profession. In general terms, these increases are based on the output expected from existing training programmes over the next few years, but they are based on the assumption that all training posts will be filled, that all of the entrants will complete their training, and that all of the graduates will seek full-time employment in the NHS. These expectations are very unlikely to be fulfilled.

Resources

The NHS Cancer Plan describes an increase in expenditure on cancer of £570 million over three years. At first glance, these resources appear to be generous and likely to exceed our ability to fill posts. In practice, however, a substantial proportion of this additional investment will be utilised by the costs of chemotherapy following National Institute for Clinical Excellence appraisal of a range of drugs that are currently being introduced. Furthermore, the allocation of the resources and their intended use was not made clear in the allocations to the NHS for 2001–02, with the result that resources were not applied to cancer as had been intended. In future years, a more directive approach will be required if cancer services are to benefit from new investment as envisaged in the NHS Cancer Plan.

Teamwork

The management of cancer through multidisciplinary teams is now an established component of all national cancer guidance. The evidence that teamwork in cancer care benefits the process and outcomes of care is limited to one or two cancers, but the technology is probably transferrable to other sites. However, merely appointing the members of the teams is not necessarily sufficient to ensure that a team approach is adopted. The *Manual of Cancer Services Standards* checklist focuses on the structure of teams and not on the ways in which they work. Examples are emerging where the functioning of the teams is at fault, but this may not be picked up by the assessment and appraisal systems that are in place. A more subtle approach is required to identify deficiencies in teamworking and to correct them.

Access

The guiding principle behind the NHS Plan and the NHS Cancer Plan is the modernisation of services. The central element of this involves speeding up access to specialist care for patients who require it. The Government has set a wide range of targets with maximum time intervals between entry and completion for each phase of the process covering diagnosis and treatment. The achievement of these targets is dependent both on recruiting to key posts in cancer care and on the organisation of services in a way that gives priority to cancer patients over people with benign disease. This adds to the tensions within hospitals in general, given that the majority of clinicians who are involved in cancer care are also responsible for other aspects of clinical services. In some ways these targets are challenging and ambitious, and the timescales for achieving them are too short. However, in other respects the targets are relatively unambitious and describe considerably longer pathways of care than would be expected in the private sector or in other countries.

Accountability

The allocation of a wide range of responsibilities to cancer networks challenges traditional lines of accountability for NHS organisations. It is paradoxical that while cancer networks are responsible for delivering the NHS Cancer Plan, it remains the statutory responsibility of health authorities, NHS trusts and primary care trusts to deliver the targets. The accountability of cancer networks themselves is unclear, although it seems likely that, along with NHS trusts and primary care trusts, they will be accountable to the new strategic health authorities. Issues relating to the employment and accountability of network staff have yet to be resolved, and relationships between the network office and its member organisations are also unclear.

The most logical way of addressing these issues is to regard the network as representing the combined interests of all of the organisations concerned, while retaining a single focus on delivering the NHS Cancer Plan and *Improving Outcomes Guidance*. All of the tensions described above are inherent in this process, and the task is exceptionally challenging.

Clinical staff are accountable to their employing organisation. However, in the context of cancer networks, such local accountability can be a further distraction from the need to make improvements in cancer care specifically. It has been suggested that some aspects of accountability and clinical governance need to be viewed on a network-wide basis, and this would cut across the responsibilities of individual sovereign organisations. This issue is also unresolved.

With the increasing move towards subspecialisation, it has also been suggested that the traditional career structure for consultants no longer serves the interests of cancer care as envisaged by the new model. For example, a clinician may well wish to contribute to the development of services in different ways during the course of their 30-year career. The five-year specialist training programme for hospital specialties may well be insufficient to prepare new consultants for the highly specialised services that they are now expected to deliver. In particular, the period after appointment as a consultant needs to be better supervised as experience is gathered in these subspecialised fields. In the later stages of a consultant's career, specific roles in teaching and clinical governance may be entertained at the expense of direct delivery of services. In the context of the existing relatively small organisations which constitute most of our NHS trusts, these changes in role are difficult to manufacture. Again, a network-wide approach would be necessary to allow consultants a choice of role at different stages of their career.

Conclusion

Taken together, the Calman–Hine Report, *Improving Outcomes Guidance* and the NHS Cancer Plan constitute a fine framework for improving cancer care in England and Wales. The challenges which they present to the NHS with regard to their implementation serve to confirm how far behind modern practice the NHS had fallen. These difficulties should be seen not as insuperable obstacles, but rather as a spur to delivery.

References

1 NHS Executive (1991) *The Health of the Nation.* NHS Executive, Leeds.

2 Department of Health (1999) *Saving Lives: our healthier nation.* Department of Health, London.

3 NHS Executive (1995) *Commissioning Cancer Services: Report of the Expert Advisory Group on Cancer.* NHS Executive, Leeds.

4 Department of Health (1997) *The New NHS: modern, dependable.* Department of Health, London.

5 Department of Health (2000) *The NHS Cancer Plan.* Department of Health, London.

6 Department of Health (2000) *The NHS Plan.* Department of Health, London.

7 NHS Executive (2000) *Manual of Cancer Services Standards.* Department of Health, London.

CHAPTER 2

The epidemiology of cancer

John Wilkinson and Anita Hatfield

General epidemiology of cancer

Cancer in the UK

About two in five people in the UK get cancer at some point in their life,[1] there are 220 000 cases of cancer (excluding non-melanoma skin cancer) diagnosed each year in England and Wales (and 26 000 cases in Scotland). An individual GP with an average list of 2000 patients will only see about eight or nine cases a year.

Mortality from cancer

Cancer is now the commonest cause of death in the UK, responsible for 25% of all deaths. The biggest killers are lung, colorectal, breast and prostate cancer, which caused 48% of all 134 000 cancer deaths in 1999.[2]

Survival from cancer

Many people will survive their cancer for at least five years. The percentage which survives for five years varies greatly with different cancers. Lung, pancreatic and oesophageal cancers kill almost all individuals who get them, whereas very few people die from skin cancer.[3] For some cancers, such as Hodgkin's disease and leukaemia of childhood, the situation has changed from there being few survivors 40 years ago to the majority surviving for at least five years.

There are variations in the numbers surviving between countries and between treatment centres. Other European countries have higher survival rates for almost all cancers than do patients in the UK.[4] If survival from cancer was as good as the European average, about 25 000 lives a year would be saved in England and Wales.[5]

Five-year survival in the UK improved for seven of the 20 common cancers between 1986–90 and 1991–93. This includes a 6–7% improvement in breast and prostate cancer, and is likely to be due to earlier detection of cancer through screening (sometimes detection of non-progressive prostate cancer) and to improved treatment (e.g. treatment of breast cancer with Tamoxifen). For some cancers the survival rates did not improve at all, and lung cancer survival rates fell, although this is thought to be due to increased registrations of patients with advanced disease.[3]

In general, there is evidence for many cancers, particularly the rarer ones, that survival is improved when specialist multidisciplinary teams give treatment to a sufficient number of cases annually.[6]

Variation in cancer between different locations

Variations in cancer within and between countries can be investigated in order to determine whether the cause is environmental, genetic, or due to lifestyle or cultural factors.

Descriptive studies

The initial studies usually focus on differences in the incidence of cancer and mortality between different areas of the world or within countries. These are generally termed ecological or descriptive studies, which may have involved cross-sectional surveys or cancer registration. The populations can then be studied in order to determine the likely causes of these variations.

The initial studies undertaken are often correlation studies showing, for example, that the incidence of cancer is lower where the intake of olive oil is higher.[7] This may not be due to olive oil *per se* but to factors that are associated with it, such as a diet high in fresh fruit and vegetables. Thus studies that link people to specific factors are required in order to confirm a cause.

Twin studies

Twin studies in which genetically identical twins can be compared with non-identical twins with regard to the incidence of cancer suggest that about 18% of cancers have a genetic component.[8] Twins reared in different countries or cultures can give further clues to causality, but such studies are necessarily rare.

Migration studies

Migration studies have been particularly helpful for teasing out those associations that are found in correlation studies. When migrants come from an area with a high incidence of a particular cancer and move to an area with a low incidence, or vice versa, then interactions between time, person and place can be tracked. If a cancer has an environmental cause, then the incidence of the disease would decrease rapidly in the cohort that was not exposed to the environmental agent. Conversely, if a disease is due to a genetic defect, the incidence would remain the same in those who did not intermarry. Diseases that had predominantly cultural causes (perhaps a type of cooking or food delicacy) would remain until the influences of the local culture had more effect than those of the immigrant's culture.

Examples of this situation come from Japanese migration to the USA. Japan has a low rate of colorectal cancer but a high rate of stomach cancer, whereas in the USA these diseases have the opposite frequencies. Over time the cancer rates in Japanese immigrants have approached those of the host country America. A change in incidence in the migrants also gives some estimate of the latent time between exposure and cancer onset.

Environmental factors

Environmental factors can increase the local incidence of cancers. One example is the presence of radon in housing, which is dependent on local geology. High radon levels in a house can increase the risk of lung cancer developing in people living there.

Clusters

Many other factors have been suspected of increasing the incidence of cancer, including nuclear power stations, electricity pylons and incinerators. The evidence for these 'causes' remains weak, and statistically is difficult to prove or disprove completely. The number of cancers in an area is likely to be affected by chance, and is very dependent on where the target area for the population is drawn. This has been described as like drawing bull's-eyes on a wall after the arrows have all been fired, so that the target is selected where most of the arrows fell. Thus clusters of leukaemia around nuclear power stations have been shown to be similar to clusters that occur in areas where there are no nuclear power stations, leading to the theory that leukaemia is more common in areas where incomers mix with well-established populations.

Prospective cohort studies

Migration studies are a specific form of cohort study. A cohort can be formed from groups that experience the same exposure to a suspected cancerous agent, and can be followed for years to discover whether that exposure has led to cancer. When this group has been compared with another which is similar to the exposed group in all respects except being exposed to this possible cancerous agent, then the excess risk in the first group can be determined. This is an excellent method of determining risk associated with a suspected agent, but it depends on first identifying the risk and the cohort, and then ensuring good follow-up of the cohort during the probably lengthy period of time when a cancer may appear. This was done most famously with the cohort of doctors which first confirmed the link between smoking and lung cancer, and subsequently the link to many other diseases. Other cohorts have been formed following disasters such as the nuclear bombs falling on Hiroshima and Nagasaki, and following the chemical disaster at Bhopal in India.

Case–control studies

Because of the long time lag in cohort studies, another type of study has frequently been used to suggest the cause of a cancer. This is termed a case–control study. In these studies cases with the disease are compared with people without the disease, and both are compared with regard to their history of exposure to the suspected carcinogens. Thus if 100 cases of mesothelioma nearly all have a documented history of exposure to asbestos, and very few of the controls have such a history, this would tend to support the hypothesis that exposure to asbestos is a cause of mesothelioma. In this type of retrospective study, the odds of developing the disease when exposed to asbestos can be compared with the odds of developing the disease when one has not been exposed to asbestos. This approximates to the relative risk of disease determined in a cohort study, but a true rate cannot be calculated. In practice it is not as easy as this, since it is difficult to avoid bias when choosing a control population that is similar to the cases except for the fact that the subjects have no disease, and when finding evidence to support the histories of both controls and cases.

Cancer in different people

Age

In general, the incidence of cancer increases with age, particularly for the common cancers such as lung and colorectal cancer, but this does not apply to all cancers. Some cancers are commonest in children. Retinoblastoma and hepatoblastoma occur in those under 1 year of age. Acute leukaemia is commonest between 2 and 4 years, and Wilms' (kidney) tumour is commonest under 5 years of age. Bone sarcoma is commonest after the age of 10 years. Hodgkin's disease can affect teenagers, but is commonest in young adults. Its incidence then declines until it rises again in those aged 50 years or over.

Sex

The incidence of cancer frequently varies between the sexes. Cancers that are specific to the genital region only occur in that sex. Prostate cancer is the second commonest cancer in men, and ovarian, uterine and cervical cancers kill over 6000 women each year.[1] Less than 1% of breast cancers occur in men, whereas this is the commonest cancer in women.

There can be obvious reasons why the incidence of some cancers varies between men and women. Lung cancer is twice as common in men because, over the previous century, men smoked at a younger age and more commonly than women. Since they have given up smoking more often than women, the lung cancer rate has decreased in men but is still rising in women.[9]

There are about 1500 registrations for cancer of the larynx each year in England and Wales, but extremely few in women. Bladder and kidney cancer is about twice as common in men as in women. Most other non-genital cancers are more common in men than in women. This is likely to be associated mainly with smoking habits and a small occupational component, and the pattern may therefore change. The exception is melanoma, which is more common in women than in men, perhaps reflecting differences in sunbathing habits between the sexes.[1]

For other variations it is more difficult to suggest reasons for the difference. Cancer of the colon has about the same incidence in men and women, but cancer of the rectum is twice as common in men. Oesophageal and stomach cancers are more common in men, and this is possibly associated with increased alcohol intake as well as smoking, but cancer of the pancreas affects both sexes equally. All of these differences can lead to possible theories about the cause of the cancer, which may be explored in cohort and case–control studies.[1]

Overall, about as many women as men develop cancer each year. The frequency distribution by age group shows that women have more cancer than men between the ages of 30 and 60 years, due to the earlier onset of breast and cervical cancer, but after that age men have more cancer than women up to the age of about 85 years.[1]

Many personal lifestyle, socio-economic, cultural and genetic factors may contribute to the risk of cancer.

Deprivation

Most cancers are more common in deprived groups, although there are exceptions such as breast and brain malignancies and melanoma of the skin. It is difficult to say whether this is because deprived groups have less healthy lifestyles or because they live in less healthy surroundings.[10]

Melanoma is thought to be more common in affluent groups, as these were the people who first developed the habit of taking summer holidays in sunny climes. Short bursts of ultraviolet light are thought to promote melanomas, whereas longer exposure such as that received by those working outdoors can cause squamous carcinomas, which are more common in agricultural workers.[11]

Occupation

Certain occupations are associated with a higher risk of cancer. This is usually due to coming into contact with materials that are now known to be carcinogenic, such as asbestos, chromium, uranium or benzenes. Some increased risk is due to associations of the job. For example, bar staff may be at risk from increased alcohol consumption and working in a smoke-filled atmosphere.

Genes

Some cancers have a genetic component. This may be suspected if there is a family history of a specific cancer occurring in younger than average individuals. Breast cancer, ovarian cancer and colorectal cancer are associated with several genes that greatly increase the risk of these cancers in people who possess these genes.

Ethnicity

Some cancers are more common in people of different race or ethnic background. This is perhaps due to a genetic component, but is often associated with factors linked to deprivation, diet, culture or lifestyle that are also linked with that ethnicity. Oral cancer in the UK is much more common in people of Indian and Pakistani origin. This is due to the habit of chewing betel nut or paan. The addition of tobacco increases the risk.

Smoking

Smoking has been implicated as a direct cause or promoter of cancer. The association was first noted for lung cancer, but smoking has since been implicated in many other cancers, including those of the bladder, cervix, oesophagus, mouth, pharynx and larynx.[12,13]

Alcohol

Alcohol has been implicated in the onset of about 3% of cancers, particularly oral, laryngeal, oesophageal and liver cancer.[14,15] The association is mainly with consumption of spirits and heavy drinking. The incidence of oesophageal cancer is particularly high in those with occupations which give them access to high-strength alcohol, such as distillery workers.

Diet

Diet is suspected of being the cause of up to one-third of cancers. It is known that a diet high in fruit and vegetables seems to protect against cancer.[16,17] Obesity is also a risk factor for some cancers. A large Danish cohort found 16% more cancers in obese individuals than in non-obese subjects. In women these were cancers of the uterus and kidney, and also breast cancer in those over 70 years of age. There were also increases in oesophageal, liver, pancreatic and colon cancers in both sexes, which suggests that these increases may be linked to alcohol and other dietary factors.[18]

Other causal factors

Many other factors have been implicated in carcinogenesis. Sunlight is a major cause of skin cancer that has already been discussed. Physical activity is thought to be protective with regard to colorectal cancer. Viruses have been implicated in some cancers, such as Epstein–Barr virus in Burkitt's lymphoma.

It can be difficult to disentangle the different influences of these factors. Some of them may interact to lead to cancer formation, while others may merely be associated with some other factor that causes cancer.

Cancer trends over time

The incidence of cancer can vary over time.

Falling incidence

The rise and fall in the incidence of lung cancer is well known. The incidence of stomach cancer is falling, and so is that of cervical cancer. These decreases are thought to be due to better diet in the case of stomach cancer, and to screening in the case of cervical cancer. The death rate from cancer in those under 75 years of age is falling.[19]

Rising incidence

The incidence of other cancers is rising. There is more oesophageal cancer, possibly associated with rising levels of alcohol intake. There is also a large increase in prostate cancer, which is thought to be due to more testing leading to an increase in the rate of diagnosis rather than a true increase in the cancer. This is confirmed by the fact that there is no increase in the number of deaths from prostate cancer despite (especially in the USA) a large increase in the number of registrations. Following the stabilisation of the screening effort, the number of cases has declined from its peak. Non-Hodgkin's lymphoma has increased both in incidence (about 3–4% annually in the USA) and in mortality. The reasons for this trend in most parts of the world are unknown, and require research to enable preventative action to be taken.[20]

Cancer registration

Data on trends are dependent on reliable population-based registration of cancer. Cancer registries that are informed of all cancers in their area with a known population can give good incidence and survival data for studying trends over time in registrations, deaths and survival from cancer. Doubts about comparative data between countries have often arisen when it has been suspected that some countries have failed to ascertain completely all cases of cancer in their area, and therefore international comparisons need to be treated with caution.

Age cohorts

Different age cohorts may experience different exposures (e.g. with regard to taking up smoking). Women who came of age during the Second World War had a much higher incidence of cervical cancer than those of earlier generations. This is thought to have been due to changes in sexual mores at that time.

Declining age-specific incidence over time

A decline in the age-specific incidence of cancer over time has been noted in the USA since 1990.[21-23] This is thought to be principally due to the declining incidence of smoking-related cancers, particularly in men. It may also reflect the healthier diets generally adopted over the preceding decades.[24] Not all areas of the world have seen this decline in incidence.[25-27] For example, this shift is not yet apparent in the UK data except for a few cancers. Trends in incidence show that the age-standardised rates between 1971 and 1996 in England and Wales have risen by 30% in females and by 16% in males.[1] Even if the UK age-specific incidence falls, there is not likely to be a reduction in the number of cancer patients who require treatment, due to the ageing of the population.

Future trends

Demographic factors

The population of the UK is ageing. In 1996 there were 1 million people aged 85 years or older, with three-quarters of these being women, and there were 10.7 million people (18%) over 65 years of age. By 2021, it is estimated that there will be 12 million people over 65 years. As the incidence of many cancers increases with age, the burden of cancer will increase as a proportion of the work of the health service.[28,29] This is despite the fact that age at diagnosis for some of the common cancers is falling, since this increase is not as fast as the increased 'greying' of the population.

Current services

Current services in the UK are hard-pressed, with long waiting times to treatment for many patients, although cancer patients are often prioritised ahead of those with other diagnoses. There are insufficient staff such as oncologists, specialist cancer nurses and therapeutic radiographers. Specialist staff are now being asked to go to more multidisciplinary meetings in order to improve cancer treatment, but this limits the time available for clinics and operating sessions. Capital infrastructure, such as linear accelerators for radiotherapy services, is difficult to fund, and many areas have inadequate available capacity and thus long waiting times for treatment. In the recent past in the UK there has been fierce controversy over different health authority policy decisions to provide expensive chemotherapy, leading to the widely criticised 'postcode lottery'. This was a particularly contentious issue with regard to the usage of taxanes as first-line treatment for ovarian cancer. Recently the National Institute for Clinical Excellence has determined that such drugs should be made available, and is therefore going some way towards eliminating these geographical variations in the availability of certain drugs.

There is evidence from Eurocare II trials that outcomes for most cancers in the UK are poorer than the average for Europe in terms of survival. Most European countries spend more of their gross domestic product (GDP) on healthcare than we do, and access to services is generally quicker than in the UK. Comparisons with Europe indicate that a lot needs to be done in order to improve cancer services in the UK. The Government has indicated that it is determined to reduce cancer deaths and provide good quality care for all, and has increased the amount of money available for cancer services. In September 2000, the UK Government published a cancer plan setting out ways in which the quality of treatment can be improved in England.[30] Improvement is certainly needed.

Epidemiology of specific cancers[31]

This section provides an overview of the epidemiology of selected individual cancers. Table 2.1 shows the provisional registrations of cancer cases in 1996. These data are derived from regional cancer registries. The ability to compile national data thus depends on the speed of the slowest. Some registries experience considerable difficulties in compiling timely data because of the mobility of their population, which is greater in larger conurbations compared with other more static areas. A series of boundary changes, and the abolition of regional health authorities in England in the mid-1990s, have led to difficulties in maintaining cancer registration across the country. As a result of these difficulties a review of cancer registries has been undertaken by Professor Charles Gillies. His report, now adopted as part of the NHS Cancer Plan, will strengthen the role of registries. However, concern has been expressed by cancer registries in the UK following publication of new guidance from the General Medical Council. This guidance was published with the intention of protecting patients'

Table 2.1:   Registrations of newly diagnosed cases of cancer in 1996 in England and Wales (provisional data)

Total registrations	Male	Female	Total
All malignant neoplasms	110 200	110 500	220 700
Oesophagus	3540	2510	6050
Stomach	6510	3630	10 140
Colon	8850	9830	18 680
Rectum	6180	4610	10 790
Pancreas	2780	3190	5970
Trachea, bronchus and lung	22 300	12 700	35 000
Melanoma	1850	2540	4390
Breast	248*	31 200	31 200
Cervix	–	2600	2600
Ovary	–	5720	5720
Prostate	18 900	–	18 900
Testis	1490	–	1490
Kidney	3060	1860	4920
Bladder	8510	3320	11 830
Brain	120	120	240
Myeloma	1550	1350	2900
Leukaemia	2860	2490	5350

Source: Office of National Statistics.[1]
* Office of National Statistics.[33]

confidentiality, and it states that doctors should not transfer individuals' details to cancer registries without their consent. Critics of this guidance say that it is unworkable and will lead to doctors no longer allowing their patients' details to be transferred to cancer registries.[32] Legislation to overcome this obstacle was passed in 2001 but has not yet been enacted.

Lung cancer

Lung cancer remains the commonest cancer in England and Wales. In 1996 there were 35 000 new registrations. Although it is rare under the age of 40 years, lung cancer is the commonest cancer in men and the second commonest cancer in women (after breast cancer). Lung cancer is gradually decreasing in incidence in parallel with earlier reductions in the level of smoking in the country. However, the balance of the disease between the sexes is changing, reflecting an increasing trend among women to smoke in the middle to latter part of the twentieth century. The incidence of lung cancer in men has been falling since the early 1980s, and was estimated to fall by a further 5% between 1993 and 1996. However, the incidence of lung cancer in women was expected to rise by 5% between 1993 and 1996. Because this condition is so common, small improvements in healthcare have quite a significant impact in terms of population health improvement. There has tended to be a nihilistic approach to the management of lung cancer, but this situation is expected to change with the publication of the national evidence-based guidelines on the management of the disease. It has been shown that by careful selection of patients significant improvements in care[34] can be achieved. Around 90% of cases of lung cancer in men and 78% of cases in women are attributable to smoking.[35] Occupational exposure is also an important factor in the epidemiology of lung cancer, and will be considered in more detail in the section on prevention.

Breast cancer

In total, 31 200 new cases of breast cancer were detected in England and Wales in 1996. The incidence of breast cancer in women remained at around 100 cases per 100 000 members of the population between 1993 and 1996. Breast cancer caused nearly 12 000 deaths in 1999, and was the commonest cause of death in women aged 35–54 years, and the commonest cause of cancer-related death in women. It is likely that lung cancer in women (11 109 cases in 1999 compared with 11 548) will soon overtake breast cancer as the leading cause of cancer death. This is already the case in Scotland, where 20.2% of cancer-related deaths in women are from lung cancer, compared with 17.5% from breast cancer.[36]

Breast cancer is predominantly a female cancer. It occurs over 100 times less frequently in men, and it affects men on average in their mid-sixties. Unlike most other cancers, breast cancer affects more women in the upper socio-economic groups, particularly women over the age of 50 years. Breast cancer is more common in the nulliparous, and in women who are obese. There is considerable geographical variation in the incidence of breast cancer around the world, with a much higher incidence in Northern Europe and Northern America compared with Africa and Asia.

After years of very little change in mortality rates, deaths from breast cancer have fallen significantly in the last ten years.[37] However, it is unclear why this is the case. It is thought likely that the national screening programme has had a major impact, although in the absence of a randomised controlled trial it is not possible to demonstrate this conclusively. Undoubtedly the attention that was given to the introduction of a national screening programme in the late 1980s provided a boost for improvement in breast cancer services. The latter were also some of the first cancer services to be subjected to detailed scrutiny following the publication of the Calman–Hine Report.[38]

The national guidelines on the management of breast cancer were the first set of guidelines to be published in 1996.[39] Breast cancer services continue to improve, and breast surgery is increasingly becoming a general surgical specialty in its own right. This is likely to lead to the creation of stand-alone breast centres which are separate from other general surgical services. Changes to the national screening programme are also anticipated in the next few years, and these are discussed in more detail in Chapter 5 on prevention.

Colorectal cancer

In 1996, almost 30 000 people were diagnosed with colorectal cancer in England and Wales. The incidence of this cancer rises rapidly after the age of 50 years. The recorded incidence is rising slightly in older age groups and falling slightly in younger adults. Rectal cancer is more common in men, whereas colon cancer is slightly more common in women. These are cancers of 'developed' countries. A small number of cases are linked to inflammatory bowel disease and familial polyposis coli. Other suggested causes have included high levels of beer consumption, and cancer of the colon has been linked to previous cholecystectomy. The aetiology of these cancers is probably dietary, involving an excess of saturated fat and lack of fibre. There is also some evidence that these cancers are linked to a sedentary lifestyle.

Gynaecological cancers

Cervix cancer

In total, 2600 new cases of invasive cervical cancer were detected in 1996, and this cancer caused 1106 deaths in 1999. Around 15% of these cases occur in individuals under 35 years of age. Cervical cancer is much more common in lower socio-economic groups, and is associated with early sexual intercourse, high number of sexual partners, human papilloma virus and smoking. These factors will be considered in more detail in Chapter 5 on prevention.

Population screening aimed at identifying cervical intra-epithelial neoplasia (CIN), which it is known can progress to cancer, has been associated with a recent decline in the incidence of cervical cancer.[40] The incidence of cervical cancer has fallen sharply since 1991 and continues to decline. There was a decrease of 23% between 1993 and 1996, and this decline is expected to continue.

Ovarian cancer

Ovarian cancer is the commonest gynaecological cancer in women. In 1996, a total of 5720 new cases were diagnosed. Ovarian cancer causes around 4000 deaths each year, and 90% of cases occur in women over 45 years of age (most are postmenopausal, with a peak incidence at 65–75 years of age). This cancer is linked with breast cancer genes (*see* Chapter 3), and is currently subject to a trial of screening.

Endometrial cancer

There are around 4000 new cases of endometrial cancer each year. This is a disease of postmenopausal women, with 75% of new cases occurring after the menopause. Only 5% of cases occur below the age of 40 years. Women with higher levels of oestrogen are at greater risk, and these include more obese women, those on unopposed oestrogen replacement therapy, women taking tamoxifen and those with polycystic ovary disease.

Vaginal cancer

This is a cancer of older women, with around 200 new registrations a year, leading to around 100 deaths a year.

Upper gastrointestinal cancers

The major upper gastrointestinal cancers are those of the oesophagus, stomach and pancreas. All of these cancers tend to have a poor prognosis as they often present at a late stage. Many of the early clinical features are similar to those of less severe conditions.

Oesophageal cancer

The main aetiological factors are alcohol and smoking, and there is also a suggested link between oesophageal cancer and poor diet. There is an increased risk in patients with coeliac disease. High rates of oesophageal cancer are seen in Central Asia and in Brittany and Normandy in France. National risks in England and Wales are among the highest in Europe, especially in women.

Stomach cancer

Death due to stomach cancer is a significant cause of cancer-related death in England and Wales, although it is on the decline. Mortality rates have decreased by 25% over the last 35 years. Stomach cancer is thought to have a mainly dietary cause. Suggested aetiological factors have included deficiencies of fresh fruit and vegetables, and it has been suggested that the decline in incidence of this cancer is linked to a change in food preservation methods from salting, pickling and smoking to refrigeration. A link between stomach cancer and *Helicobacter pylori* has been demonstrated. An increased risk of stomach cancer is seen in individuals with blood group O and those who are exposed to ionising radiation. It has been noted that the position of stomach cancers has been shifting from the pylorus to the gastro-oesophageal junction, and there is concern that with better treatment of benign upper gastrointestinal problems with H_2 (histamine receptor) antagonists, this could mask the early stages of stomach cancer. This means that doctors need to consider the possibility of stomach cancer in patients with any persisting upper gastrointestinal symptoms lasting for over six weeks, and gastroscopy is indicated in anyone over 55 years of age in whom such symptoms persist. Around 90% of stomach cancers occur in those aged 55 years or over, so the risk of this cancer below this age is small compared with the large number of people with stomach pains.[41]

Pancreatic cancer

Cancer of the pancreas is often rapidly fatal, with a median survival time of about 3–4 months in England.[42] The overall 5-year survival rate is 2%.[2]

Smoking is known to be a causative factor. It is estimated that up to 40% of pancreatic cancers in men and 20% of these cancers in women can be attributed to this cause. In 1996 there were almost 6000 new cases of pancreatic cancer, with 5926 deaths registered in 1999. The age-standardised rates have declined since 1987 in England and Wales from 11.3 per thousand in men and 8.2 per thousand in women to 9.8 and 7.7, respectively. The crude rates are almost equal in men and women (11.8 and 12, respectively, in 1993), despite the fact that the disease is more common in men of any age. The incidence of the disease rises steeply with age from 2.3 in men aged 40–44 years (1.2 in women) to 106.8 in those over 85 years of age (81.5). As there are more elderly women in the population, twice as many women experience and die from the disease as men.

Urological cancers

Prostate cancer

In 1996, a total of 18 900 men were diagnosed with prostate cancer in the UK. The incidence of prostate cancer rises steadily with age. However, only 12% of cases are clinically apparent before the age of 65 years. Prostate cancer is the third commonest cause of cancer-related death in men, with 8689 deaths in 1993. In 1993, prostate cancer was the second commonest cancer in men, its incidence exceeding that of colorectal cancer. However, the mortality rate fell in 1996 and 1997 after a consistent rise during the 1980s and 1990s. There is an increased tendency to diagnose prostate cancer with the growing use of prostate-specific antigen (PSA) testing. The natural history of prostate cancer is poorly understood, making its treatment problematic and possibly in some cases unnecessary.

Bladder cancer

There were 11 830 new cases of bladder cancer in 1996 in England and Wales. Bladder cancer is almost three times more common in men than in women. This cancer has been associated with smoking and occupational exposure to certain chemical substances (*see* Chapter 5 on prevention).

Renal cancer

There were 4920 new cases of renal cancer in 1996, and 2700 patients died of the disease in 1999. The 5-year survival rate is about 30%. This cancer is almost twice as common in men as in women. The incidence increases with age from 5.1/100 000 in males aged 40–44 years (2.1/100 000 in women) to a peak of 59/100 000 in men aged 75–79 years (28.1/100 000 in women aged 80–84 years). Smoking is thought to account for about 20% of cases of renal cancer. This cancer is twice as common in those who smoke 40 or more cigarettes per day.[43]

It has been suggested that renal calculi increase the risk of renal cancer, but a Swedish cohort found only an increased risk of renal pelvis, ureter and bladder cancer, particularly on the same side as the stone.[44]

Testicular cancer

There were 1490 new cases of testicular cancer in 1996. This cancer accounts for 1% of male cancers. It most commonly occurs in young men aged 18–45 years, and it is the commonest cancer in men aged 20–34 years. Testicular cancer is four and a half times more common in Caucasian males. It is associated with undescended testicles and irradiation. Several epidemiological studies have described an increasing incidence in adult men over time,[45] and it has been suggested that the main reason for this is the secular trend towards earlier puberty.[46]

Haematological cancers and lymphomas

Hodgkin's disease[47]

The overall incidence of Hodgkin's disease is 2.4 per 100 000 in the UK. It is one of the commonest malignancies in young people. It is more common in young adults with higher socio-economic status, and in older adults with lower socio-economic status. There is an overall male predominance, with a male : female ratio of 1.5 : 1, the male excess being most pronounced in childhood. Certain types (non-sclerosing) account for the young adult peak. Other types increase with age. For example, cases of Hodgkin's disease non-sclerosing (HDNS) are increasing in incidence. It has been suggested that Hodgkin's disease is a contagious disease, but this has never been substantiated. It has also been suggested that Hodgkin's disease behaves in a similar way to paralytic poliomyelitis. For both of these diseases the age peak in incidence increases as living standards increase, and for both there is an increased risk with higher social class and reduced family size. It has been suggested that Hodgkin's disease is a rare manifestation of a common infection, and this view is supported by the observation that the risk of Hodgkin's disease is higher in people who have had a low incidence of childhood infections.[48]

Non-Hodgkin's disease

The risk factors for non-Hodgkin's disease (or non-Hodgkin's lymphoma; NHL) include a family history of leukaemias and lymphomas and a history of infectious mononucleosis, and occupational exposure to wood dusts and glues has also been suggested. NHL is the fifth leading cause of death in men and the seventh leading cause in women. The average age at diagnosis is 42 years. The incidence of NHL is continuing to increase. Evidence from the National Cancer Institute and the Surveillance, Epidemiology and End Results (SEER) has shown increases of 4% and 3% in men and women, respectively. Some of this increase is due to improved diagnostic techniques, changes in disease classification and the increase in AIDS-related lymphomas, but most of the increase is unexplained. Viruses are thought to play a major role in some subtypes of lymphoma (especially Epstein–Barr and HTLV-1), and with improved molecular techniques, more viruses which may play a part in NHL are likely to be identified. Some immunodeficiencies have been shown to predispose individuals to NHL.[49]

Leukaemias

Leukaemia is classified into four main diseases, each of which is considered below.

Acute myeloblastic leukaemia (AML)

The rates of AML vary widely. In Europe there is a fourfold variation in incidence, with the highest rates being reported in Scotland, Switzerland, Italy and Denmark. The causes of AML are unclear, but some evidence has been published linking AML as a sequel to chemotherapy or radiotherapy for other primary malignancies. Other risk factors have also been suggested, including exposure to benzene, cigarette smoking and a family history of leukaemia or lymphoma. Non-random cytogenetic changes have been detected in 50% of cases. The incidence of AML decreases slightly after early childhood and then increases with age. In later years AML is more common in men than in women.

Chronic myeloid leukaemia (CML)

The incidence of CML is usually slightly higher in men than in women. The highest rates have been reported in US blacks in Alameda, non-Kuwaitis in Kuwait, and in Western Australia. There is some evidence linking incidence with radiation, but it is much less clear for other suggested causes (e.g. exposure to benzene). Like AML, CML may follow treatment of primary malignancies with radiotherapy or chemotherapy. Most if not all cases of CML have a chromosomal abnormality, whether it be the Philadelphia chromosome (a 9:22 translocation) or other abnormalities. Therefore there is a strong possibility that these chromosomal abnormalities have some pathogenic importance.

Acute lymphoblastic leukaemia (ALL)

The published rates for lymphoblastic leukaemia vary sevenfold throughout the world. Rates in India are reported to be low. Risk factors include prior chromosomal defects such as Down's syndrome, fetal exposure to X-rays, and a history of miscarriages in the mother. Other aetiologies have been suggested, including parental exposure to certain chemicals, exposure to chloramphenicol, and viral infections. Most patients with ALL do not appear to have any predisposing condition or exposure to potential risk factors. ALL peaks in incidence in childhood at the age of 2–3 years. There is no evidence of sex differences in younger age groups, but there is some evidence of a male excess in adolescents and in patients over the age of 60 years.

Chronic lymphatic leukaemia (CLL)

Most registrations of lymphoid leukaemia are CLL in individuals over the age of 50 years. The highest reported rates of CLL are in Israel, Australia, Europe and North America, with notably low rates being reported in Japan and Asian countries. Risk factors are similar to those for NHL rather than the other leukaemias. CLL affects more males than females.

References

1   Office of National Statistics (1999) Registrations of cancer diagnosed in 1993–1996, England and Wales. *Health Stat Quart.* **4**: 59–70.

2   Office of National Statistics (2000) Death registrations in 1999: cause England and Wales. *Health Stat Quart.* **6**: 64–70.

3   Office of National Statistics (2000) Cancer survival in England and Wales, 1993–1996. *Health Stat Quart.* **6**: 71–80.

4   Coeburgh J, Sant M, Berrino F and Verdecchia A (1998) Survival of adult cancer patients in Europe diagnosed from 1978–1989. EUROCARE II Study. *Eur J Cancer.* **34**: 2137–278.

5   Sikora K (1999) Cancer survival in Britain. *BMJ.* **319**: 461–2.

6   Selby P, Gillis C and Haward RA (1996) Benefits from specialised cancer care. *Lancet.* **348**: 313–18.

7   Stoneham M, Goldacre M, Seagroatt V and Gill L (2000) Olive oil, diet and colorectal cancer: an ecological study and a hypothesis. *J Epidemiol Commun Health.* **54**: 756–60.

8   Verkasalo PK, Kaprio J, Koskenvuo M and Reeves G (1999) Genetic predisposition, environment and cancer incidence: a nationwide twin study in Finland, 1976–1995. *Int J Cancer.* **83**: 743–9.

9   Shopland DR (1995) Tobacco use and its contribution to early cancer mortality with a special emphasis on cigarette smoking. *Environ Health Perspect.* **103** (**Supplement**): 131–42.

10 Greenwald HP, Borgatta EF, McCorkle R and Polissar N (1996) Explaining reduced cancer survival among the disadvantaged. *Millbank Quart.* **74**: 215–38.

11 Lear JT, Tan BB, Smith AG *et al.* (1998) A comparison of risk factors for malignant melanoma, squamous cell carcinoma and basal cell carcinoma in the UK. *Int J Clin Pract.* **52**: 145–9.

12 McLaughlin JK, Hrubec Z, Blot WJ and Fraumeni JF Jr (1995) Smoking and cancer mortality among US veterans: a 26-year follow-up. *Int J Cancer.* **60**: 190–3.

13 Engeland A, Anderson A, Haldorsen T and Tretli S (1996) Smoking habits and risk of cancers other than lung cancer: 28 years follow-up of 26 000 Norwegian men and women. *Cancer Causes Control.* **7**: 497–506.

14 Turner C and Anderson P (1990) Is alcohol a carcinogenic risk? *Br J Addiction.* **85**: 1409–15.

15 International Agency for Research on Cancer (1988) Alcohol drinking. Epidemiological studies of cancer in humans. *Monogr Eval Carcin Risk Hum.* **44**: 153–250.

16 Hertog MG, Bueno-de-Mesquita HB, Fehily AM, Sweetnam PM, Elwood PC and Kromhout D (1996) Fruit and vegetable consumption and cancer mortality in the Caerphilly Study. *Cancer Epidemiol, Biomarkers Prev.* **5**: 673–7.

17 Potter JD (1997) Diet and cancer: possible explanations for the higher risk of cancer in the poor. *International Agency for Research on Cancer (IARC) Scientific Publications (Lyon).* **138**: 265–83.

18 Moller H, Mellemgaard A, Lindvig K and Olsen JH (1994) Obesity and cancer risk: a Danish record-linkage study. *Eur J Cancer.* **30A**: 344–50.

19 Dickinson HO (2000) Cancer trends in England and Wales. *BMJ.* **320**: 884–5.

20 Hartge P, Devessa SS and Fraumeni JF (1994) Hodgkin's and non-Hodgkin's lymphoma. *Cancer Surveys.* **19–20**: 423–53.

21 McKean-Cowdin R, Feigelson HS, Ross RK, Pike MC and Henderson BE (2000) Declining cancer rates in the 1990s. *J Clin Oncol.* **18**: 2258–68.

22 Wingo PA, Ries LAG, Rosenberg HM and Edwards BK (1998) Cancer incidence and mortality 1973–1995: a report card for the US. *Cancer.* **82**: 1197–207.

23 Ries LAG, Wingo PA, Miller DS *et al.* (2000) The annual report to the nation on the status of cancer, 1973–1997, with a special section on colorectal cancer. *Cancer.* **88**: 2398–424.

24   Merrill RM (2000) Measuring the projected impact of lung cancer through lifetime and age-conditional risk estimates. *Ann Epidemiol.* **10**: 88–96.

25   van Leer EM, Coeburgh J and van Leeuwen FE (1999) Trends in cancer incidence and mortality in The Netherlands: good and bad news. *Ned Tijdschr Geneeskd.* **143**: 1502–6.

26   Swerdlow A, dos Santos Silva I, Reid A, Qiao Z, Brewster DH and Arrundale J (1998) Trends in cancer incidence and mortality in Scotland: description and possible explanations. *Br J Cancer.* **77 (Supplement 3)**: 1–16.

27   Hoel DG, Davis DL, Miller AB, Sondik EJ and Swerdlow A (1992) Trends in cancer mortality in 15 industrialised countries 1969–1986. *J Natl Cancer Inst.* **84**: 313–20.

28   Bey P (2000) Future trends in oncology. *Support Care Cancer.* **8**: 98–101.

29   Sharp L, Black RJ, Muir CS, Gemmell I, Finlayson AR and Harkness EF (1996) Will the Scottish Cancer Target for the year 2000 be met? The use of cancer registration and death records to predict future cancer incidence and mortality in Scotland. *Br J Cancer.* **73**: 1115–21.

30   Department of Health (2000) *The NHS Cancer Plan: a plan for investment, a plan for reform.* Department of Health, London.

31   Swerdlow A and dos Santos Silva I (1993) *Atlas of Cancer Incidence in England 1968–85.* Oxford University Press, Oxford.

32   Brown P (2000) Cancer registries fear imminent collapse. *BMJ.* **321**: 849.

33   Office of National Statistics (1999) *Registrations of Cancer Diagnosed in 1993, England and Wales.* The Stationery Office, London.

34   NHS Executive (1998) *Improving Outcomes in Lung Cancer.* NHS Executive, London.

35   Health Education Authority (1998) *The UK Smoking Epidemic: deaths in 1995.* Health Education Authority, London.

36   (1999) *Cancer Registration Statistics Scotland 1986–1995.* Scottish Cancer Intelligence Unit (SCIU) Information and Statistics Division (ISD), NHS Scotland (http://www.show. scot.nhs.uk/isd/scottish_health_statistics/subject/canceregistra/index.htm).

37   McPherson KM, Steel CM and Dixon JM (1995) Breast cancer – epidemiology, risk factors and genetics. In: JM Dixon (ed.) *ABC of Breast Diseases.* BMJ Books, London.

38   Expert Advisory Group on Cancer (1995) *A Policy Framework for Commissioning Cancer Services: a report by the Expert Advisory Group on Cancer to the Chief Medical Officers of England and Wales.* HMSO, London.

39   NHS Executive (1996) *Improving Outcomes in Breast Cancer.* NHS Executive, London.

40   van Winjgaarden WJ, Duncan ID and Hussain KA (1995) Screening for cervical neoplasia in Angus: 10 years on. *Br J Obstet Gynaecol.* **102**: 137–42.

41   Department of Health (2000) *Referral Guidelines for Suspected Cancer.* Department of Health, London (http://www.doh.gov.uk/pub/docs/doh/guidelines.pdf).

42 Northern and Yorkshire Cancer Registration and Information Service (2000) *Cancer Treatment Policies and Their Effects on Survival: pancreas.* Key Sites Study 4. NYCRIS, Leeds.

43 McLaughlin JK, Hrubec Z, Heineman EF, Blot WJ and Fraumeni JF Jr (1990) Renal cancer and cigarette smoking in a 26-year follow-up of US veterans. *Pub Health Rep.* **105**: 535–7.

44 Chow WH, Lindblad P, Gridley G *et al.* (1997) Risk of urinary tract cancers following kidney or ureter stones. *J Natl Cancer Inst.* **89**: 1453–7.

45 Forman D and Moller H (1994) Testicular cancer. *Cancer Surveys.* **19–20**: 323–41.

46 Moller H, Jorgensen N and Forman D (1995) Trends in incidence of testicular cancer in boys and adolescent men. *Int J Cancer.* **61**: 761–4.

47 Jarrett RF (1992) Hodgkin's disease. *Balliere's Clin Haematol.* **5**: 57–79.

48 Gutensohn N and Cole P (1977) Epidemiology of Hodgkin's disease in the young. *Int J Cancer.* **19**: 595–604.

49 Palackdharry CS (1994) The epidemiology of non-Hodgkin's lymphoma: why the increased incidence? *Oncology (Huntingt).* **8**: 67–73.

CHAPTER 3

Genetics and cancer

John Wilkinson and Carol Chu

Genetics and prevention of cancer

Approximately one in three people in the UK will develop cancer during their lifetime. The vast majority (90–95%) of cancers occur by chance as the end result of many different factors, such as lifestyle and environment. If cancer occurs in this way, then the relatives of the affected individual are not at any greater risk than anyone else who is exposed to the same environmental factors. However, in a minority of cancers there is a strong genetic element which will lead to a tendency to develop cancer in that individual. The genetic element may be due to either a single-gene disorder or genetic polymorphisms.

Single-gene disorders are conditions which are caused by alterations (mutations) in a particular gene. Mutations are disease causing if they either alter an amino acid or produce a shortened or truncated protein. In some conditions there is only one gene that will cause the clinical picture (e.g. familial adenomatous polyposis coli; FAP), but in others the clinical picture can be due to changes in one of several genes (e.g. breast and ovarian cancer can be caused by mutations in one of two genes – *BRCA1* and *BRCA2*). However, in any particular family only one gene causes the condition.

Genetic polymorphisms are normal variations in a gene sequence occurring in the population at large. Conventionally, gene alterations are considered to be polymorphisms if they occur in 1 in 100 normal individuals in the population. These polymorphisms do not cause disease *per se*, but they may alter an individual's response to environmental factors.

Single-gene disorders

Rare familial cancer syndromes, such as Li-Fraumeni syndrome (LFS) and familial adenomatous polyposis coli (FAP), have been recognised for many years.

These conditions are inherited in an autosomal-dominant manner, so children of an affected individual have a one-in-two risk of having the condition. In these syndromes there is nearly inevitable development of cancer at a young age in individuals with the tendency, unless preventative treatment is given.

More recently it has become apparent that although most 'common' cancers, such as breast or colorectal cancer, are the end result of multiple factors, around 5–10% of cancers are due to a genetic tendency. In these cases, the tendency is inherited in an autosomal-dominant fashion. However, in most cases the tendency bestows a high risk of developing cancer but it is not inevitable. Families with a genetic predisposition to cancer exhibit the following characteristics:

- cancer occurs at a younger age than expected
- there are multiple cases of the same or related cancers in the family
- there may be more than one primary cancer in an individual.

It is vitally important that those families who are at genetic risk are identified, because individuals from such families have a very much higher risk of developing cancer than the rest of the population, and may develop the cancer at an unexpectedly young age (e.g. colorectal cancer occurring during the twenties). Recognising these individuals results in targeting of resources to those who are at highest risk, and prevents unnecessary and potentially harmful screening for those who are not at high genetic risk. It will also allow a surveillance programme to be initiated for that individual, and will help to identify individuals who might benefit from preventative strategies. Table 3.1 shows neoplasms for which genetic testing is possible at the moment.

If gene testing for cancer predisposition in a family is to be offered, it is necessary first to identify the disease-causing mutation in an affected member of the family. In some cancer syndromes there are common mutations, such as in MEN2. In others there are common mutations in particular ethnic groups, but for the general population there are many different possible mutations. For instance, there are over 200 different mutations that have been described in *BRCA1* and *BRCA2*. Some of these may be unique to a particular family (a private mutation). However, there are common mutations seen in the Ashkenazi Jewish population, with a high frequency of these mutations in the population.

Gene testing is not fully automated and is extremely labour intensive. An analysis of a single family may necessitate several hundred separate reactions being set up by a scientist. Such testing therefore takes a considerable period of time (six to twelve months would not be unusual to identify a family mutation). Subsequent testing of other family members would be much quicker, since it would only require searching for that particular mutation. In the future, as technology improves, gene testing will become more automated and therefore faster, so that a higher rate of throughput will be possible.

Table 3.1: Cancer predisposition syndromes for which mutation testing is available in the UK

Condition	Features	Gene name
FAP	Multiple colonic polyps/colorectal cancer, desmoid, sebaceous cysts, epidermoid cysts, multiple duodenal polyps/periampullary carcinoma	APC
Von Hippel–Lindau disease	Central nervous system haemangioblastomas, retinal angiomata, renal cysts/carcinoma, pancreatic cysts/carcinoma, phaeochromocytoma	VHL
Li-Fraumeni syndrome	Sarcomas, breast cancer, brain tumours, adrenocortical carcinoma, leukaemia	P53
MEN2	Medullary thyroid carcinoma, parathyroid adenoma, phaeochromocytoma	RET
MEN1	Pituitary adenomas, parathyroid adenoma, pancreatic tumours	MENIN
Gorlin disease	Basal cell carcinomas, cardiac fibromata, medulloblastoma, congenital anomalies, lamellar calcification of falx cerebri	PTCH
Breast/ovarian cancer	Breast cancer, ovarian cancer, colorectal cancer, prostate cancer	BRCA1, BRCA2
Cowden's disease	Breast cancer, intestinal hamartomas, cerebellar gangliocytoma, cutaneous and mucosal papillomas	PTEN
HNPCC	Carcinomas of colon, endometrium, ovaries, stomach, hepatobiliary system and urinary tract system	hMLH1, hMSH2, PMS1, PMS2
Atypical melanoma mole	Dysplastic naevi, malignant melanoma	CDKN^{p16}, CDK4

FAP, familial adenomatous polyposis coli; MEN, multiple endocrine neoplasia; HNPCC, hereditary non-polyposis coli.

Once a gene mutation has been found in an affected family member, then unaffected, at-risk individuals can be offered testing as well (predictive testing). If they do not have the mutation then they will not be at increased risk of cancer and will not require extra surveillance, but if they do have the mutation then they will be at high lifetime risk of developing cancer, and will need either extra surveillance or preventative treatment.

Mutation detection techniques will not detect 100% of mutations, and this, as well as the fact that there may be more than one gene which can produce the same clinical picture, means that *not* finding a mutation in an affected individual would not exclude a genetic predisposition in that family.

Mutation detection for cancer tendency is currently available in most NHS regional DNA laboratories. However, commercial patenting of genes may mean that such testing by diagnostic laboratories may become restricted in the future, or the cost of testing may increase if laboratories have to pay for licences to be allowed to perform testing in particular genes.

For individuals, the decision to undergo predictive testing for cancer predisposition syndromes can be extremely difficult for the following reasons:

- uncertainty about the development of cancer, since the presence of the mutation will mean that the individual is at high risk, but may not mean that the development of cancer is inevitable
- the psychological implications of knowing about the high risk of developing cancer without a guaranteed strategy for reducing that risk
- uncertainty about the best medical management for individuals at high risk
- implications for children or for reproductive decisions
- implications for insurance.

A family history of cancer does sometimes influence decisions with regard to insurance. A gene test that will actually predict that an individual is at very high risk of developing cancer may make it more difficult or costly or even impossible to obtain certain types of insurance. In order to consult on the difficult topic of genetic tests and insurance, the Department of Health has established a Genetics and Insurance Committee (GAIC) consisting of experts representing scientific, medical, insurance and patients' viewpoints. The GAIC aims to establish precisely which tests are relevant to insurance. The Association of British Insurers has developed a code of practice with regard to gene testing and insurance. This code acknowledges that the applicant for insurance has a choice as to whether or not to take genetic tests. The code does not allow insurers to insist that someone takes a genetic test as a condition of offering them insurance, but if such a test has been taken then the test result must be given to the insurer. The GAIC has the final say in the relevance to insurance of specific genetic test results. Genetic test results need not be shown to insurers in new applications for life insurance up to £100 000 that are directly linked with a new mortgage. From October 2001, the UK insurance companies agreed a five year voluntary moratorium such that genetic tests will not be taken into account unless the policy for life insurance exceeds £500 000.

Genetic counselling in these circumstances is therefore vitally important in order to enable individuals to make fully informed choices and to support them through the testing procedure. The uptake of predictive testing for breast cancer predisposition when such counselling is offered is approximately 50%. There would be concerns that individuals who are tested in a commercial setting would not receive such counselling.

The Health Services Circular HSC 1998/031 for England and Wales on Cancer Genetic Services has suggested a model for triaging families which involves the filtering of such families first by general practitioners in primary care, secondly by surgeons/oncologists at cancer unit level, and finally by the regional genetics service at cancer centre level. There are various suggestions as to how this should be implemented, such as a computer program used in primary care setting which aims to identify families who should be referred for further advice.[1] The NHS Cancer Plan (2000) is in favour of this model for primary care working in conjunction with Macmillan Cancer Care. There are also other models that may be useful.

Genetic polymorphisms and cancer risk

Apart from the dominant cancer syndromes, as mentioned previously, there are genetic polymorphisms which appear to be important in the development of cancer. Some polymorphisms may affect an individual's response to various environmental exposures. It has been suggested that women with a particular (arginine) polymorphism at codon 72 of the *p53* gene may have a higher risk of developing human papilloma virus (HPV)-associated cervical cancer than women with other polymorphisms.[2] It has also been suggested that slow acetylators who carry the N-acetyltransferase 2 slow acetylation polymorphism and who smoke are at higher risk of bladder cancer (35%) than are fast acetylators who smoke (13%).[3] However, there are conflicting results from different studies. Researchers are investigating the role of polymorphisms in certain genes, such as those for cytochrome P450 (*CYP1A1* and *CYP2E1*) and glutathione-S-transferase (*GSTM1* and *GSTT1*) in several different cancer types, including cancer of the cervix uteri, lung, oral cavity, bladder, prostate and oesophagus.

In addition to this gene–environment interaction in the development of cancer, genetic polymorphisms may be important in prognosis. It has been suggested that the number of CAG trinucleotide repeats in the androgen-receptor gene is shorter in women with more aggressive breast cancers.[4] This same CAG repeat may be important in prostate cancer progression, since a short repeat appears to be a risk factor for recurrence in men who would otherwise be deemed to be at low risk of recurrence.[5]

In the future, these genetic polymorphisms may well be used to try to prevent cancer in those at higher risk by modification of behaviour such as smoking. They may also guide the clinician by suggesting more aggressive treatment in certain individuals with cancer who carry certain polymorphisms.

Prevention of cancer in individuals at high genetic risk

If a family has been shown to have a genetic tendency to cancer, it is frequently possible to detect the gene mutation responsible for the familial tendency. If the gene mutation is characterised, then predictive testing can be offered to at-risk family members to ascertain whether they also have inherited the mutation. If an individual does not have the family mutation, then their risk is reduced to the same as that for the rest of the population. However, if they do have the mutation, they will be at very high lifetime risk of cancer. There are various different options available for attempting to prevent cancer.

Surgery

Prophylactic surgery can be offered to try to prevent cancer in these high-risk cases. In many familial cancer syndromes such surgery has been shown to prevent cancer. For example, more than 99% of individuals with gene mutations in the *APC* gene, which causes FAP, will develop multiple colonic polyps from mid-childhood onwards. Since there are so many polyps, there is inevitable progression to cancer, which on average occurs around the age of 40 years. Total colectomy when polyps appear will prevent the development of colorectal cancer.

This prophylactic surgical approach is used not only when there is an extremely high risk of cancer, but also when the cancer itself is difficult to detect and treat. For example, in multiple endocrine neoplasia, there is a high risk of individuals with a gene mutation in the *RET* oncogene developing medullary thyroid cancer. This cancer has an excellent prognosis if it is treated at an early stage (100% ten-year survival rate for stage 1) with total thyroidectomy, but a poor prognosis if it is detected at later stages (20.7% ten-year survival rate for stage IV).[6] Therefore prophylactic thyroidectomy is suggested for children under the age of ten years with the gene mutation.

In other familial cancers the evidence for prophylactic surgery is less clear. In familial breast cancer, prophylactic surgery is likely to reduce the risk by 90% or more.[7] However, it is unclear what type of surgery is optimal and whether the level of risk reduction is the same for individuals with known gene mutations. In other familial cancer syndromes, such as pancreatic cancer, renal cancer and stomach cancer, high morbidity and significant mortality risks may make the prospect of prophylactic surgery unacceptable for many surgeons and patients.

In the future, as surgical techniques improve, mortality and morbidity will decrease and there will be improvements in transplant surgery. It may then be acceptable to have prophylactic surgery to remove the at-risk organ and replace it. Although tissue cloned from the individual would not be usable, it is possible that tissue could be cloned from a close, unaffected relative for this use.

Chemoprevention

Chemoprevention is the prevention of cancer by treatment with chemical agents such as drugs, hormones, vitamins, foodstuffs or minerals. Chemoprevention is an attractive strategy for individuals who are known to be at high genetic risk of developing cancer. There have been more than 15 observational studies, using case-controlled, nested case–control and prospective designs, which have investigated the relationship between aspirin/non-steroidal anti-inflammatory drugs (NSAIDs) and colorectal cancer. The findings of the majority of these studies have suggested that NSAIDs are effective in reducing adenoma formation and lowering the incidence of colonic carcinoma.[8] A total of 14 uncontrolled case series and four small randomised trials have looked at the role of sulindac in subjects with FAP. These reports suggest that adenomata can regress on treatment, but that complete regression is unlikely. However, it is still unclear which agents are the best ones, what dose should be used and for how long they should be used. Cyclo-oxygenase inhibitors have shown substantial cancer prevention in animals and adenoma regression in humans, although reductions or delays in cancer incidence have not yet been demonstrated.[9] There are ongoing studies examining the efficacy of aspirin or resistant starch (CAPP-1)[10] or the selective COX-2 inhibitor celecoxib in FAP.

Similar work has been piloted in hereditary non-polyposis coli (HNPCC), a familial syndrome in which multiple colonic polyps occur giving a high (80% lifetime risk) of developing colorectal cancer as well as risks of endometrial, ovarian, stomach, urinary tract and biliary tract cancers. Three phase II studies have been published looking at the role of calcium carbonate in HNPCC.[9] An international randomised controlled study of the use of aspirin or resistant starch (CAPP-2) in HNPCC is also ongoing.

The role of such chemoprevention is less clear in other cancer syndromes, such as breast cancer. There is controversy over the use of agents such as tamoxifen in different trials. Four trials have been performed, and others are still ongoing. Three of the trials have shown good results, with the largest one showing an approximately 50% reduction in breast cancer risk in the short term. However, there are significant side-effects, such as risk of thromboembolism and endometrial cancer.[11] Other drugs such as raloxifene (a selective oestrogen receptor modulator) are currently being assessed in clinical trials.

Other drugs and naturally occurring substances have also shown some promise with regard to possible prevention of cancer. Indole-3-carbinol, which occurs in high concentration in cruciferous vegetables such as broccoli and cabbage, has been shown to reduce mammary cancer in rodents, probably by reducing substrate availability to C16 alpha-hydroxysterone, which is an oestrogen metabolite.[12] Green tea, which contains polyphenolic antioxidants, has also been found to be protective against cancer in many animal-tumour bioassays.[13] Studies involving these high-risk cohorts may have applications to the prevention of cancer in a sporadic setting as well.

The future

The Human Genome Project aims to determine the entire sequence of the human genome and is due to be completed in 2003. At present, 38 000 genes have been confirmed and a further 115 000 gene elements have been identified. However, even though a sequence may be known, the function of the genes within that sequence will not be known, and further research will be needed to determine the function of the genes identified. Undoubtedly there will be more cancer genes identified in the future, some of which will be associated with a very high risk of cancer (highly penetrant genes) and some of which will be associated with a lower risk of cancer (less penetrant genes).

As new genes are discovered and their function is elucidated, there will be improved understanding of the process of cancer development. This in turn will lead not only to better therapies but also to prevention of cancer in individuals with an increased susceptibility, for whatever reason.

References

1 Emery J, Walton R, Coulson A, Glasspool D, Ziebland S and Fox J (1999) Computer support for recording and interpreting family histories of breast and ovarian cancer in primary care (RAGs): qualitative evaluation with simulated patients. *BMJ.* **318**: 32–6.

2 Storey A, Thomas M, Klita A *et al.* (1998) Role of a p53 polymorphism in the development of human papilloma-virus-associated cancer. *Nature.* **393**: 229–33.

3 Marcus PM, Hayes RB, Vineis P *et al.* (2000) Cigarette smoking, N-acetyltransferase 2 acetylation status, and bladder cancer risk: a case series meta-analysis of a gene-environment interaction. *Cancer Epidemiol Biomarkers Prev.* **9**: 461–7.

4 Yu H, Bharaj B, Vassilikos EJ, Giai M and Diamandia EP (2000) Shorter CAG repeat length in the androgen receptor gene is associated with more aggressive forms of breast cancer. *Breast Cancer Res Treat.* **59**: 153–61.

5 Nam RK, Elhaji Y, Krahn MD *et al.* (2000) Significance of the CAG repeat polymorphism of the androgen receptor gene in prostate cancer progression. *J Urology*. **164**: 567–72.

6 Modigliani E, Cohen R, Campos J-M *et al.* and the GETC study group (1998) Prognostic factors for survival and for biochemical cure in medullary thyroid carcinoma: results in 899 patients. *Clin. Endocrinol.* **48**: 265–73.

7 Hartmann LC, Schaid DJ, Woods JE *et al.* (1999) Efficacy of bilateral prophylactic mastectomy in women with a family history of breast cancer. *NEJM*. **340**: 77–84.

8 Decensi A and Coata A (2000) Recent advances in cancer chemoprevention, with emphasis on breast and colorectal cancer. *Eur J Cancer*. **36**: 694–709.

9 Hawk E, Lubert R and Limburg P (1999) Chemoprevention in hereditary colorectal cancer syndromes. *Cancer*. **86**: 2551–63.

10 Burn J, Chapman PD, Mathers J *et al.* (1995) The protocol for a European double-blind trial of aspirin and resistant starch in familial adenomatous polyposis: the CAPP study. Concerted Action Polyposis Prevention. *Eur J Cancer*. **31A**: 1385–6.

11 Cuzick J (2000) A brief review of the current breast cancer prevention trials and proposals for future trials. *Eur J Cancer*. **361**: 1298–302.

12 Osbourne MP (1999) Chemoprevention of breast cancer. *Surg Clin North Am*. **79**: 1207–21.

13 Mukhtar H and Ahmad N (1999) Green tea in chemoprevention of cancer. *Toxicol Sci*. **52**: 111–17.

CHAPTER 4

Cancer screening

John Wilkinson

Introduction

The UK National Screening Committee defines screening as a public health service in which members of any defined population, who do not necessarily perceive themselves to be at risk of, or are already affected by, a disease or its complications, are asked questions or offered a test in order to identify those individuals who are more likely to be helped than harmed by further tests or treatment to reduce the risk of that disease or its complications.[1]

Screening which is aimed at apparently healthy individuals is different to clinical practice where individuals are seeking advice and help. Although screening has the potential through early diagnosis to save life or to improve the quality of life, it also has the potential to harm. Such harm may be caused by a false-negative result (a person wrongly reported as not having a condition) or a false-positive result (a person wrongly reported as having a condition). Screening tests are not 100% accurate, and false-positive and false-negative results are an intrinsic part of the test (its specificity and sensitivity). Screening may reduce the risk of developing a condition or its complications, but it does not guarantee that an individual does not have or will not develop the disease.

Population screening programmes in the UK

Screening programmes consist of complicated clinical, administrative, educational, quality and monitoring elements. The screening test is only one part of the programme. Therefore evidence of the effectiveness of a screening test alone is not sufficient for the introduction of a new screening programme. Wilson and Junger formulated a series of criteria for screening for disease.[2] The UK National

Screening Committee further developed these criteria in 1998[3] to take into account the more rigorous requirements for evidence of effectiveness, as well as the greater concern among both the general population and professionals about the adverse effects of screening. The criteria look at factors concerning the following:

- the condition being screened for (its epidemiology, natural history and primary prevention)
- factors concerned with the test itself (its simplicity, accuracy, safety and acceptability, and the further investigation required of people with a positive test result)
- the treatment of the condition (the evidence of better outcomes of early treatment, and the evidence base for the appropriate treatment to be offered)
- the screening programme (reduction of morbidity and mortality, acceptability of the whole programme, benefit, harm and opportunity cost, the quality systems, the facilities and staff in place, and information available to participants).

The National Screening Committee

In 1996 the UK National Screening Committee[3] was established to advise Ministers on the following:

- the case for introducing new population screening programmes
- implementing new screening technologies of proven effectiveness requiring controlled and managed introduction
- the case for continuing, modifying or withdrawing existing population screening programmes.

The National Screening Committee is charged with establishing practical mechanisms to oversee the introduction of new screening programmes and their implementation in the NHS. It also monitors the effectiveness and quality assurance of screening programmes. In 1996, the NHS was instructed not to introduce new screening programmes until the National Screening Committee had reviewed their effectiveness.

The National Screening Committee currently oversees two nationwide cancer screening programmes (cervical and breast cancer) and has a UK colorectal cancer screening pilot under way. In 1997 it advised on population screening for prostate cancer and concluded that, at that time and with the technology currently available, there was no evidence of benefit from a population screening programme.[4]

In England the breast screening and cervical screening programmes also each have a National Advisory Committee (which includes the UK representatives) which offers advice to the National Screening Committee and NHS Executive in England. There is also a National Co-ordinating Office for the cancer screening programmes in England which is responsible for developing systems and guidelines to ensure a high-quality screening programme throughout the country, to identify important policy issues and help to resolve them, and also to improve communications within the programme and with participants.

In addition, each English region has a quality assurance centre for the breast and cervical cancer screening programmes which is accountable to the Regional Director of Public Health, as well as links with the National Co-ordinating Office.

At the time of writing, the relationship of the National Screening Committee and these structures to the National Institute for Clinical Excellence (NICE) and the Commission for Health Improvement (CHI) is unclear. NICE is charged with establishing the evidence base for interventions and making recommendations to the NHS in England and Wales, and the CHI has an investigatory and monitoring role for health services.

The cervical cancer screening programme

The NHS cervical screening programme was established in 1988 when all health authorities introduced computerised call and recall systems. Cervical screening is a method of preventing cancer by detecting and treating precancerous changes in the cervix. The programme aims to reduce both the number of women who develop invasive cancer and the number of women who die from it. All women between the ages of 20 and 64 years are eligible for a cervical smear test at least once every five years. Health authorities invite women who are registered with a general practitioner to use a computerised call and recall system. The system also keeps track of any follow-up investigation and, if all is well, recalls the women for screening at a due date in the future. The programme screens almost 4 million women in England each year, and 84% of these women have been screened within the previous five years. The NHS Plan[5] has recently announced that, over the next few years, liquid-based cytology will be introduced into the NHS. This is a new technology for preparing the smear samples to increase their accuracy and reduce the number of inadequate cervical smear tests taken. Automation of the smear-reading process is currently also being examined within the programme. Such technology will assist and improve the smear-reading process and the efficiency of the service.

The breast screening programme

Breast screening is a way of detecting breast cancers when they are very small. Those which are detected at an early stage are easier to treat and respond to a wider range of treatments. The first stage of screening is an X-ray examination of each breast (a mammogram). The aim of the NHS breast screening programme, which was set up in 1988, is to reduce the number of women who die from breast cancer. Women aged between 50 and 64 years are routinely invited for breast screening every three years, and women aged 65 years and over are encouraged to make their own appointments. As a result of a pilot that looked at the practical implications and resources which would be needed if older women were routinely invited for screening, the upper age limit for routine invitations to the NHS screening programme will shortly be increased to 70 years.[5] Women under 50 years of age are not offered routine screening. A national trial was started in 1991 to investigate what benefit, if any, is gained by screening women under 50 years of age, and that trial will run for 15 years.[6] The current programme invites women for a repeat screening every three years. A trial has recently been completed which looked at the benefits of offering screening annually instead of on a three-yearly basis. This trial is expected to report in the near future.[6] About 20% of the cancers detected by the screening programme are ductal carcinoma *in situ* (DCIS). In these cancers, the cancer cells have not spread through the walls of the breast ducts to the rest of the breast tissue or beyond to become an invasive cancer. Not all DCIS progresses to become invasive cancer. There is currently a United Kingdom Coordinating Committee for Cancer Research (UKCCCR) trial in progress to determine the best means of treating such cancers.

Screening difficulties

The challenge for cancer screening programmes in 2000 and beyond is to achieve the outcomes reported by enthusiasts involved in initial randomised controlled trials of screening, in a routine service setting on any cold wet Friday afternoon.

The cancer screening programmes have experienced several well-publicised incidents which have been the subject of investigation, including the Inverclyde report on cervical screening in 1993,[7] the Kent and Canterbury report on cervical screening[8] and the Exeter report on breast screening.[9] The Nuffield Institute[10] identified the common issues arising from these incidents, which included the following:

- inadequate numbers of well-trained staff
- the need to integrate screening services into mainstream NHS management processes

- the need to clarify the management structures and accountability within screening programmes
- the need for well-defined national standards
- the virtues of the current quality assurance system
- the benefits of multidisciplinary peer review.

The modernising agenda for screening programmes in the next decade includes the following:

- the further development of quality systems and standards
- addressing the staffing issues facing the programmes
- finding effective methods of providing information for those invited for screening
- where the evidence base justifies it, introducing new high-quality cancer screening programmes (e.g. colorectal cancer screening).

Quality systems

Recent incidents associated with screening programmes[7–9] have left the public, politicians and professionals bruised and upset by failures in the services. Quality systems will identify errors, and these need to be investigated and the lessons learned fed back to the programme. Screening programmes should look at building in compensation for patients involved in such incidents without them having to seek redress through the courts. This would help to recognise the realities and limitations of cancer screening.

The Nuffield Report on quality management for screening[10] recommends that screening programmes should have clear frameworks of objectives, standards and guidance. The continued development of national standards in the cancer screening programmes should be evidence based with input from the professional groups, staff, users and the health departments. There should be continuous quality improvement with standards being updated in the light of new evidence and experience. The measurement of performance needs to be collated and analysed in a consistent manner across the whole programme. This is to enable problems to be identified and managed earlier. There should be clarity of management structures and accountability, as well as open systems for measuring the performance against national standards. Performance management should be at a distance from those who are providing the service in order to maintain some objectivity. The quality management should focus on the competence of the whole system as well as the competence at an individual level. Screening programmes should operate within a culture of learning and not

blame. Users of the service should be involved in developing the quality management systems. This will require work in the next few years at national, regional
and local levels. In England, the commissioning of the local cancer screening
programme is through a named individual operating at least at district level.
With the advent of primary care trusts in England, it is important that the commissioning of the cancer screening programmes rests at a population level large
enough to enable appropriate measurement of performance.

Staff

Motivated and appropriately trained staff are the key to successful programmes.
The performance management of the programme must be developed in the context of a supportive learning environment, rather than a threatening one.
When the only feedback on performance that staff receive is through the head-
lines in the local evening paper about another scandal, morale drops and staff
recruitment and retention become much more difficult. There are shortages of
trained staff in both national cancer screening programmes at present. Screening programmes must develop better career pathways, training, pay and conditions for those involved in the service. The introduction of new technologies
(e.g. automation of cervical smear reporting) may help to relieve workload pressures on staff. Alternative approaches to the problem include considering
breaking down the current professional boundaries and skill mixes. This may
be achieved by training staff to take on roles that have not traditionally been
theirs (e.g. radiographers reading breast-screening films).

Informed choice

Raffle[11] has commented that 'Screening has distorted public belief. In a desire
for good population coverage, we have said screening is simple, effective and
inexpensive. In truth, it is complex, of limited effectiveness and very expensive.
The simple message "cervical cancer is preventable" means to the lay person
every death is someone's fault.' A major challenge for existing and new screening programmes has to be how they effectively convey information about the
benefits and harmful effects of screening to members of the population so that
the latter are giving their informed consent when they take up an offer of
screening. The proposed colorectal cancer screening programme, if it is implemented across the country, will save many lives, but may also kill some apparently healthy individuals during the screening/diagnostic process.

Professionals, and increasingly the public, know that even in the best-run screening programmes the nature of the screening test will result in false-negative results. Coupled with tests which require great skill to interpret subtle changes, this means that cancers have been missed by screening programmes in the past and will continue to be missed in the future.

The information that has been provided about screening programmes in the past has addressed the benefits of screening positively, but has been less forthcoming and explicit about the potential harm that can be caused. Coulter[12] has criticised screening programme materials for emphasising the benefits and glossing over the risks. The cancer screening programmes are now starting to address how individuals who have been offered screening can receive full and accurate information about the screening test and its sequelae.[1]

Screening programmes have adopted a paternalistic approach to what it is felt the population can understand and cope with, concerned that information about potential harm will stop people taking up an offer of screening.[13] Further research is needed on how best to give people the evidence-based information necessary to enable them to make an appropriate choice.[13] The screening programmes look to primary care professionals to provide most information to patients. Ways need to be developed to keep them informed with up-to-date information and provide them with the time they require to discuss these issues with their patients.

In cervical screening, general practitioners are currently financially rewarded for achieving uptake targets. Perhaps the rewards need to shift towards the quality of information given to potential participants so that these individuals have all of the appropriate information necessary to make an informed choice as to whether or not to take up the screening offer.

New cancer screening programmes

Colorectal cancer is the second largest cause of cancer deaths in the UK. Research has shown that screening can help to reduce death rates by diagnosing and treating bowel cancer at an early stage. It is predicted that deaths from bowel cancer could decrease by 15% as a result of screening. Nationally, screening for bowel cancer could save approximately 2500 lives each year. The NHS has commissioned a pilot scheme to screen for colorectal cancer in two sites, one in England (Coventry and Warwickshire) and the other in Scotland (Dundee).[14] Starting in 2000, for two years men and women aged between 50 and 69 years in the pilot site areas are being offered screening for bowel cancer using a faecal occult blood test. This test looks for tiny amounts of blood in a sample of bowel motion. If the pilot scheme is successful, it is anticipated that this will then become a new national cancer screening programme.

The Imperial Cancer Research Fund (now Cancer Research UK) is undertaking a further trial using flexible sigmoidoscopy as the screening test.

Prostate cancer fulfils some of the criteria required of a disease that might be managed by population screening. In men aged 50–60 years, rectal examination and prostate-specific antigen testing will detect clinically suspicious areas within the prostate. However, it is not known which of the prostate cancers, which are known to be present in 30–40% of men aged over 60 years, will be detected. Only a small proportion of cancers that are known to be present become clinically evident, and more men die with prostate cancer than because of it. There is also uncertainty as to how effective aggressive local treatments are in altering the natural history of the disease. It is unclear whether screening would be followed by a reduction in morbidity and mortality. A screening effect has been observed in the USA, with an increase in incidence and a decrease in the proportion of men with metastases.[15] The National Screening Committee is developing a prostate cancer risk management programme to offer further advice to people who are anxious about the disease. The most urgent evidence that is required concerning prostate screening is evidence of the effectiveness of different treatment strategies.

Ovarian cancer is the fourth commonest cause of cancer death among women in the UK. At present, this cancer does not meet the criteria set out by a national screening committee for a screening programme. A trial of ovarian cancer screening (the UK Collaborative Trial of Ovarian Cancer Screening) is due to start soon which is intended to involve 200 000 women in the UK over a period of ten years. Of those who will be offered screening, half will be screened with ultrasound and half with the blood test CA 125. Information from this trial will be used to help to decide whether ovarian cancer screening should be included as a national programme in the future.

Lung cancer is a very common disease, and in its earliest stages up to 70% of cases can be cured by surgery. Despite this, the overall prognosis of lung cancer is very poor. Four randomised trials in the 1970s failed to show a significant reduction in mortality from screening. Recently the Early Lung Cancer Action Project group in New York and Montreal reported initial results on the usefulness of annual computed tomography scanning compared with chest radiography in heavy smokers over the age of 60 years. This is rekindling interest in looking at trials of lung cancer screening.[16,17]

References

1 National Screening Committee; www.nsc.nhs.uk

2 Wilson JMG and Jungner G (1968) *Principles and Practice of Screening for Disease*. Public Health Paper No. 34. World Health Organisation, Geneva.

3 Department of Health (1998) *First Report of National Screening Committee. Health departments of the UK*. Department of Health, London.

4 Department of Health (1997) *Population Screening for Prostate Cancer*. Department of Health, London.

5 Department of Health (2000) *The NHS Plan*. Department of Health, London.

6 National Office of NHS Cancer Screening Programmes (2000) *NHS Breast Screening Programme*. National Office of NHS Cancer Screening Programmes, Sheffield; www.cancerscreening.nhs.uk/breastscreen/

7 The Scottish Office (1993) *Report of the Inquiry into Cervical Cytopathology at Inverclyde Royal Hospital, Greenock*. HMSO, Edinburgh.

8 Department of Health, NHS Executive South Thames Regional Office (1997) *Review of Cervical Screening Services at Kent and Canterbury Hospitals NHS Trust by a Panel Chaired by Sir William Wells, Chairman, NHS Executive South Thames*. Department of Health, London.

9 Calman K and Hine D (1997) *Breast Cancer Services in Exeter and Quality Assurance for Breast Screening: Report to the Secretary of State*. Department of Health, London.

10 Balmer S, Bowens A, Bruce E *et al.* (2000) *Quality Management for Screening. A Report for the National Screening Committee*. Nuffield Institute for Health, Leeds.

11 Raffle A (1998) New tests in cervical screening. *Lancet*. **351**: 297.

12 Coulter A (1998) Evidence-based patient information. *BMJ*. **317**: 225–6.

13 Austoker J (1999) Gaining informed consent for screening. *BMJ*. **319**: 722–3.

14 National Office of NHS Cancer Screening Programmes (2000) *NHS Colorectal Cancer Screening Pilots*. National Office of NHS Cancer Screening Programmes, Sheffield; www.cancerscreening.nhs.uk/colorectal/

15 Neal DE, Leung HY, Powell PH *et al.* (2000) Unanswered questions in screening for prostate cancer. *Eur J Cancer*. **39**: 1316–21.

16 Henschke CI, McCauley DI, Yankelevitz DF *et al.* (1999) Early Lung Cancer Action Project: overall design and findings from baseline screening. *Lancet*. **354**: 99–105.

17 Smith IE (1999) Screening for lung cancer: time to think positive. *Lancet*. **354**: 86–7.

CHAPTER 5

Preventing cancer

John Wilkinson

Box 5.1: Advice on lifestyle factors to reduce cancer risk[1]

- Do not smoke.
- Take regular exercise.
- Do not be sexually promiscuous.
- Avoid prolonged exposure to direct sunlight.
- Avoid hepatitis B and C risks.

Framework for prevention[2]

Prevention is traditionally classified into primary, secondary and tertiary prevention.

Primary prevention occurs when attempts are made to reduce or remove the cause of a disease. In cancer, the best example of primary prevention is reducing the risk of cancer through smoking reduction strategies. Identifying and removing cancer-causing substances (carcinogens) from the environment would also be classified as primary prevention. This may occur in the working environment, e.g. exposure to aromatic amines from occupational sources (such as rubber manufacturers, the cable industry and the production of dyestuffs concerning the link to bladder cancer).

Secondary prevention encompasses the early detection and treatment of disease. The purpose of secondary prevention is to increase the likelihood of a cure. As well as detecting established disease early on and encouraging patients to detect disease before it progresses, it also includes the screening programmes. Screening is considered in detail in Chapter 4.

Tertiary prevention aims to reduce the impact of established disease. Surgery, chemotherapy and radiotherapy may be used to attempt to prevent the disease

Table 5.1: Percentage of cancer deaths attributable to different factors

Factor	Percentage of all cancer deaths	
	Best estimate	Range
Tobacco	30	25–40
Alcohol	3	2–4
Diet	35	10–70
Food additives	<1	−5–2
Reproductive and sexual behaviour	7	1–13
Occupation	4	2–8
Pollution	2	<1–5
Industrial products	<1	<1–2
Medicines and medical procedures	1	0.5–3
Geophysical factors	3	2–4
Infection	10?	1–?
Unknown	?	?

Source: Doll and Peto.[3]

from recurring, although inevitably there is some overlap with secondary prevention.

Scope for prevention

It has been suggested that around 80% of all cancers are caused by non-genetic factors and are therefore preventable (*see* Table 5.1).[3,4] With recent advances in genetic understanding even this figure may now be an underestimate.

Inequalities and cancer

In England and Wales, Acheson in his report on inequalities in health described growing differences across the social spectrum in mortality from cancer in men and women, particularly in relation to lung cancer and smoking. There is a higher prevalence of smoking in the lower socio-economic groups. In 1996, 29% of men and 28% of women smoked, but the variation across socio-economic groups ranged from 12% of men (11% of women) in professional classes to 41% of men (36% of women) in unskilled manual occupations. More people in the more advantaged groups stop smoking, with cessation rates showing an increase from 25% to 50% since 1973.[5]

Reduction of risk factors

Smoking

For some time it has been clearly established that cigarette smoking is by far the most preventable factor in the causation of many cancers. This link was first established in relation to lip and mouth cancer, and then in relation to lung cancer in the 1950s.[6] Table 5.2 shows the burden of cancer on UK citizens estimated by the Health Education Authority, based on 1995 mortality data.

Cigarette smoking had become common in the UK in the first part of the twentieth century. Around 80% of men and 40% of women smoked, but until the early 1950s the link between cigarette smoking and lung cancer was largely unrecognised.[8]

National statistics now show that in 1998, 27% of adults aged 16 years or over smoked in England (28% of men and 26% of women). The prevalence of smoking is higher for people in manual groups than for those in non-manual groups (32% vs. 21%). In total, 69% of smokers wanted to give up. In 1999, 9% of children aged 11–15 years were reported to smoke, with girls smoking more than boys (10% vs. 8%).[9]

A recent study has concluded that people who stop smoking can avoid most of the risk of lung cancer, and that stopping before middle age avoids more than

Table 5.2: Estimated percentages and numbers of deaths from cancer attributable to smoking in the UK (based on 1995 mortality data)[7]

Condition	Percentage of deaths from the condition attributable to smoking in 1995		Number of deaths from the condition attributable to condition in 1995		
Cancer	*Men*	*Women*	*Men*	*Women*	*Total*
Lung	90	73	21 000	9500	30 500
Throat and mouth	74	47	1500	400	1900
Oesophagus	71	62	2900	2600	5500
Bladder	48	17	1700	300	2000
Kidney	41	5	700	100	800
Stomach	35	10	1700	300	2000
Pancreas	21	25	600	800	1400
Unspecified site	34	7	2400	500	2900
Leukaemia	19	10	200	100	300

90% of the attributable risk. The extent to which young people today become persistent smokers will affect mortality rates in the middle and second half of the twenty-first century.

Smoking has decreased over the last 50 years due to a number of factors. In 1998, the UK Government published a new strategy, aimed at reducing smoking, called *Smoking Kills*.[10] This strategy set out action in the following key areas:

- EU ban on tobacco advertising
- tobacco tax kept above the rate of inflation
- £100 million aimed at those under 16 years, adults (especially those who are disadvantaged) and pregnant women.

The taxation of cigarettes has played a major part in the strategy to reduce smoking. Chancellors of the Exchequer in England have in successive years raised the taxation on cigarettes in the UK above the rate of inflation.

Health education and health promotion interventions have a key role to play in reducing smoking, but are notoriously difficult to evaluate. However, there are increased opportunities to influence health promotion efforts to reduce the level of smoking in the community, with attention being paid to smoking in schools, at a local level (e.g. targeted efforts in primary care), at a regional level (e.g. in health action zones) and nationally as part of national strategies (e.g. *Saving Lives: Our Healthier Nation*).

The reduction in the number of places where smoking is permitted has also had an important effect in both limiting the opportunities to smoke and protecting the non-smoking public.

The National Cancer Plan for England[11] states that local targets for smoking reductions will be set, and interventions will be made explicit for the 20 health authorities with the highest smoking rates. In addition to the national *Smoking Kills* targets of reducing smoking in adults from 28% to 24% by the year 2010, new targets are to be set to address inequalities, with a target reduction in manual workers from 32% (the 1998 figure) to 26% by 2010.

Evidence of the health impact of passive smoking has been accumulating over the last 20 years. Passive smoking has been linked to lung cancer in a number of studies. Hackshaw and colleagues analysed 37 previously published studies and concluded that the lifelong excess risk of non-smokers living with a smoker was 24%.[12] Further evidence came from a study conducted in 12 European centres in seven European countries, in which a small increased risk of lung cancer was found in non-smokers who worked in a smoky environment or who lived with a spouse who smoked.[13]

In addition, passive smoking has a number of other effects on health in addition to its effect on cancer.[14,15]

Diet and cancer

- Up to 80% of bowel and breast cancer may be preventable by dietary change.
- Diet contributes to varying extents to the risk of many other cancers, including cancer of the lung, prostate, stomach, oesophagus and pancreas.
- In general, fruit, vegetables and fibre have a protective effect, whereas red meat and processed meat increase the risk of developing cancer.
- Other lifestyle/environmental factors that increase the risk include smoking, alcohol and overweight.
- Risk is decreased by physical activity.
- There is no evidence that vitamin supplements help to prevent cancer.[1]

Cancer is caused by an abnormality of cellular DNA, usually due to one or more mutations. The vast majority of cases of cancer in the UK are sporadic rather than hereditary. The dietary impact on cancer is therefore thought to be due either to producing protective mechanisms (apoptosis) or to producing carcinogens. Some animal studies have also given weight to this argument. There is currently no evidence relating diet to DNA damage, although this is an area of substantial research at the present time.

Recently, the UK Government in its cancer plan for England[11] set out two main approaches to improving the diet in the population with a view to reducing cancer. These initiatives are as follows:

- a national five-a-day programme – the aim being to increase access to fresh fruit and vegetables in order to encourage the general population to increase its intake to five portions of fruit or vegetables a day
- a national school fruit scheme – a free piece of fruit will be made available each school day to schoolchildren aged between 4 and 6 years.

Breast cancer

Hormones have been shown to have an impact on the onset of breast cancer (*see* pages 65–6 in this chapter), and diet is known to have an effect on some of these factors. For example, high-energy intake and obesity hasten the onset of menarche, whereas it may be delayed by a high intake of fibre. Serum levels of oestrogen are related to weight, and they fall in postmenopausal women who lose weight, although the same effect does not occur in premenopausal women. Postmenopausal women have up to a twofold increased risk. Meat and alcohol have both been shown to increase the risk of breast cancer, although dietary fat itself has not been shown to be a major risk factor.[16]

The reasons for the link between breast cancer and meat are unclear. However, laboratory experiments have shown a link between certain chemicals that are produced during the cooking of meat and mammary cancer in rodents.[17]

Other dietary constituents which are thought to be weakly anti-oestrogenic include low intake of vegetables and non-starch polysaccharides.

Lung cancer

The main cause of lung cancer is smoking. It has been reported that patients who develop lung cancer eat less fruit and vegetables than do members of the healthy population. This is thought to be due to the active chemotherapeutic effect of β-carotene. However, several trials of β-carotene have failed to confirm this hypothesis.

Colorectal cancer

It has been well established that fibre and vegetables reduce the risk of colorectal cancer, probably mainly due to the effect that fibre has in producing a regular bulky stool. Stool weight is low in countries with a high incidence of colorectal cancer.[18] People who eat more red meat (e.g. beef, pork and lamb) and processed meat (e.g. sausages, hamburgers and bacon) are at higher risk of colorectal cancer. High intake of meat is thought to cause cancer in a variety of ways, both by the cooking process and by increasing the dietary residues that enter the large bowel. Two phenotypes have been described for dealing with chemicals that are produced in the cooking process, namely fast and slow acetylators. Fast acetylators have an increased risk of developing polyps and large bowel cancer.[19]

Other factors have been implicated in colon cancer, including obesity, iron, calcium and some compounds found in vegetables (e.g. folate, phyto-oestrogens, sulphur-containing compounds and antioxidants).

Stomach cancer

The incidence of cancer of the stomach has been falling throughout the world. This is thought to be due to the decrease in salt intake and the replacement of traditional methods of food preservation (which often involved large amounts of salt) by refrigeration.

Individuals who eat five servings of fruit or vegetables a day are estimated to approximately halve their risk of stomach cancer.

Oesophagus

The main risk factor for cancer of the oesophagus in the Western world is smoking. Alcohol consumption in the range 40–100 grams per day produces a three- to eightfold increase in risk, with synergistic effects with smoking.[16] In well-nourished populations, a high fruit and vegetable intake is protective, whereas in undernourished populations, this increases the risk. Smoked foods are also thought to confer an additional risk.

Pancreas

A link between diet and pancreatic cancer has been suggested but not substantiated. Red meat appears to be associated with an increased risk while fruit and vegetables, vitamin C and fibre may confer some protection. Smoking is the major non-dietary risk factor known.

Prostate cancer

The incidence of prostate cancer has been increasing in recent years. High levels of consumption of red meat and fat are associated with a modest risk. Consumption of vegetables (especially salads and tomatoes) is associated with a lower risk.[20]

Gynaecological cancers

Body weight increases the risk of endometrial cancer.[21] Cancer of the cervix is found less frequently in women who consume large amounts of vegetables, folic acid and antioxidant vitamins.

Box 5.2: Advice on dietary factors to reduce cancer risk[1]

- Eat plenty of fruit and vegetables (at least five portions a day).
- Eat plenty of cereal foods (especially unprocessed).
- Maintain ideal body weight (i.e. body mass index 20–25) and avoid fatty foods.
- Eat red meat and processed meat in moderation (less than 140 g/day).
- Avoid high-dose vitamin supplements.
- Consume alcohol in moderation (maximum of 2 units per day for women and 3 units per day for men).
- Avoid highly salted and mouldy foods.

Radiation

Ionising radiation

Radiation is said to be ionising when it has the potential to accelerate electrons. Exposure to ionising radiation is ubiquitous. The first indications that radiation might have an adverse effect on health were reported in the 1930s when cases of bone cancer were detected in young women whose occupation involved painting watch faces with luminescent paint.[22]

Considerable epidemiological evidence was gathered from the populations of Nagasaki and Hiroshima following the explosion of the atomic bombs in 1945. There is now evidence that ionising radiation can cause cancer in any organ in which cancers occur naturally.[23]

The overall cancer risk from ionising radiation is small but preventable. Exposure from medical uses (including screening) must be kept to a minimum, particularly in vulnerable people (e.g. pregnant women and young children). Exposure in industry also needs to be kept to a minimum.

Radon gas

It has been shown that radon gas may account for 1 in 20 cases of lung cancer in the UK. Radon is a naturally occurring gas, and although concentrations remain relatively low, it can accumulate inside houses. Parts of the UK are affected differentially, the worst affected areas being in Devon and Cornwall, and parts of Somerset, Derbyshire and Northamptonshire also being affected to a lesser degree. Local authorities around the country in radon-affected areas have been undertaking publicity campaigns and arranging free monitoring in conjunction with the National Radiological Protection Board. Where high levels of radon are found, it is possible to increase ventilation in order to remove the harmful gas. There are also plans to modify building regulations in areas with a high radon concentration.[24]

Non-ionising sunlight

For some time health professionals have described a link between sunlight and ill health. This has not always been the case, and sunlight was regarded as an effective treatment for tuberculosis in the past.[25] The main health promotion message has been to reduce exposure to sunlight in order to prevent the development of malignant melanoma. However, the link between sunlight and melanoma is by no means simple. A systematic review of case–control studies confirmed that there was a link between intermittent exposure to the sun, sunburn and malignant melanoma. However, this effect was not demonstrated in people who were exposed to sunlight as a result of their occupation. Indeed, in this group a reduced risk was demonstrated.[26] The other factor which needs to be considered in preventative strategies is the rarity of the disease. Melanoma caused 697 deaths in men and 698 deaths in women in England in 1995. Therefore it has been suggested that population-based campaigns aimed at reducing exposure to sunlight are only likely to have small effects. Some authors have suggested that more effective preventative strategies may include raising awareness of the condition and improving access to treatment. Other links with sunlight have been suggested. For example, a link between the incidence of non-Hodgkin's lymphoma and sunlight has been proposed. However, such a link has not been confirmed.[27] Exposure to sunlight is directly linked to basal-cell skin cancers.

Non-ionising mobile phones (Stewart Report)

Because of the interest in the health effects of mobile phones, the Minister for Public Health in England commissioned an expert group to review the possible health effects of mobile phones. The Stewart Report on Mobile Phones and Health by the Independent Expert Group on Mobile Phones, chaired by Sir William Stewart, was published in May 2000.

This report concluded that 'the balance of evidence does not suggest that mobile phone technologies put the health of the general population of the UK at risk'. The group did state that there was some preliminary evidence that outputs from mobile phones did have subtle biological effects, but they did not conclude that these had an adverse impact on health. However, the Stewart Report recommended that the use of mobile phones by children for non-essential calls should be discouraged.

Non-ionising electromagnetic radiation

There have been a number of suggestions that the presence in the environment of electromagnetic radiation from power transformers and from microwave transmitters is linked to cancer. However, no substantive evidence of links has been found.

Drugs and cancer

Oral contraceptives

There has been found to be no increase in breast cancer in women who have used oral contraceptives in their late twenties to space pregnancies. However, use of the pill for four years or longer by younger women almost certainly increases the risk of premenopausal breast cancer.[28] Large studies have shown that the slight increase in risk in pill takers gradually decreases over ten years, after which there appears to be no risk. However, McPherson has more recently suggested that because these studies were conducted some time ago when patterns of contraceptive use were different, these findings may not apply at the present time and the risks may be underestimated.

Hormone replacement drugs

It has been shown that hormone replacement therapy can have beneficial effects in reducing the incidence of ischaemic heart disease and osteoporosis. However, studies of the use of unopposed oestrogen have shown that the risk of breast cancer is increased by a factor of 50% after 10–15 years of use.

Occupational and environmental factors and cancer

It is difficult to estimate the proportion of deaths from cancer that are attributable to occupational and environmental factors. The best-known risk factor is asbestos and its association with lung cancer, which is said to account for 50% of all occupational cancer deaths.[29]

Asbestos

Asbestos has been recognised for several decades as a cause of lung cancer and mesothelioma of the lung and peritoneum.[30] As a consequence, in the 1980s there was prolonged activity aimed at reducing exposure to asbestos in the workplace. Attention later turned to non-occupational exposure. A number of cases of mesothelioma were reported in the spouses of asbestos workers. Studies have been undertaken in an attempt to determine whether there is an excess risk in the population living in asbestos mining areas, but to date no such excess has been demonstrated.[31]

Other occupational hazards

As well as specific substances that are associated with cancer (some examples of which are listed in Table 5.3), a number of industrial processes are also known to increase the risk of cancer (*see* Table 5.4).

Other environmental carcinogens

It is difficult to quantify the effect of potential environmental carcinogens such as pollution for the general population. The best estimates suggest that air pollution in large conurbations may have accounted for up to 5% of lung cancer and 1% of all cancer deaths for the generations that are most exposed (i.e. those in the 1950s and 1960s).[33,34] It has been suggested that environmental

Table 5.3: Chemicals and groups of chemicals that are causally associated with cancer in humans, and to which the main type of exposure is of occupational origin

Chemical or group of chemicals	Target organs
4-Aminobiphenyl	Bladder
Arsenic and certain arsenic compounds	Skin, lung (liver, lymphopoietic system)
Asbestos	Lung, pleura, peritoneum (gastrointestinal tract, larynx)
Benzene	Leukaemia
Benzidine	Bladder
Bis(chloromethyl) ether and technical-grade chloromethyl ether	Lung
Certain mineral oils	Skin (respiratory tract, bladder, gastroinestinal tract)
Chromium and certain chromium compounds	Lung (nasal cavity, gastrointestinal tract)
Coal tars	Skin
Erionite	Pleura
Mustard gas	Respiratory tract
Beta-naphthylamine	Bladder
Nickel and nickel compounds	Nasal sinus, lung (larynx)
Shale oils	Skin (colon)
Soots	Skin, lung
Talc containing asbestos fibres	Lung
Vinyl chloride	Liver (lung, brain, lymphatic and haematopoietic system, gastrointestinal tract)

Source: Vannio.[32]
Suspected associations are shown in parentheses.

Table 5.4: Industrial processes that are causally associated with cancer in humans

Industrial process	Target organs
Aluminium production	Lung
Auramine production	Bladder
Boot and shoe manufacture	Bone marrow, nasal sinus (bladder)
Coal gasification (older process)	Skin, lung (bladder)
Coke production	Skin, lung (kidney)
Furniture manufacture (wood dusts)	Nasal sinus
Isopropyl alcohol manufacture	Nasal sinus (larynx)
Iron and steel founding	Lung
Manufacture of magenta	Bladder
Rubber industry	Bladder, leukaemia (stomach, lung, skin)
Underground haematite mining (exposure to radon)	Lung

Source: Vannio.[32]
Suspected associations are shown in parentheses.

pollutants may potentiate the effects of tobacco, making smokers more vulnerable to carcinogens other than tobacco.[35]

The constant presence of existing and new potential carcinogens highlights the need for continued vigilance through the Health and Safety Executive and ongoing epidemiological studies in occupational groups.

Infections and cancer

Worldwide, the most important infectious causes of cancer are hepatitis B and C viruses, which are both associated with hepatic cancer.[35] Internationally, liver cancer is the fifth commonest cancer in the world, accounting for 5% of cancers in both sexes.[36] Vaccination is available for hepatitis B in some European countries, but in the UK it is currently restricted to health workers, including medical students and those in high-risk occupations.

Human papilloma virus has long been known to be a cause of cervical cancer.[37] Foreman reported that *Helicobacter pylori* infection is the major cause of chronic gastritis, which is a major risk factor for stomach cancer.[38]

There have been reports that various viral agents are responsible for lymphomas. However, such relationships remain poorly understood, with the exception of those between the Epstein–Barr virus and Burkitt's lymphoma, and also between herpes virus 8 and Kaposi's sarcoma.[39] Kaposi's sarcoma is also linked to the HIV virus.

Useful websites

Action on Smoking and Health	www.ash.org.uk
Department of Health	www.doh.gov.uk
Oncolink – University of Pennsylvania	www.oncolink.upenn.edu
NHS Cancer Plan	www.doh.gov.uk/cancer
NHS Plan	www.nhs.uk/nhsplan

References

1 Cummings JH and Bingham SA (1998) Diet and the prevention of cancer. *BMJ.* **317**: 1636–40.

2 Donaldson LJ and Donaldson RJ (2000) *Essential Publ Health Med.* **3**: 101–68.

3 Doll R and Peto R (1981) *The Causes of Cancer.* Oxford University Press, Oxford.

4   Doll R (1986) *Possibilities for the Prevention of Cancer*. The Royal Society, London.

5   Acheson D (1998) *Independent Inquiry into Inequalities and Health*. Office for National Statistics, London.

6   Doll R (1998) Uncovering the effects of smoking: historical perspective. *Stat Methods Med Res*. **7**: 87–117.

7   Health Education Authority (1998) *The UK Smoking Epidemic: deaths in 1995*. Health Education Authority, London.

8   Peto R, Darby S, Deo H, Silcocks P, Whitley E and Doll R (2000) Smoking, smoking cessation, and lung cancer in the UK since 1950: combination of national statistics with two case–control studies. *BMJ*. **321**: 323–29.

9   Department of Health (2000) *Statistics on Smoking England 1998*. Department of Health, London.

10 Department of Health (1998) *Smoking Kills*. Department of Health, London.

11 Department of Health (2000) *The NHS Cancer Plan: a plan for investment, a plan for reform*. Department of Health, London.

12 Henshaw AK, Law MR, and Wald NJ (1997) The accumulated evidence on lung cancer and environmental tobacco smoke. *BMJ*. **315**: 980–88.

13 Boffetta P (1998) Multicenter case–control study of exposure to environmental tobacco smoke and lung cancer in Europe. *J Natl Cancer Inst*. **90**: 1440–50.

14 National Cancer Institute (1999) *Health Effects of Exposure to Environmental Tobacco Smoke. The Report of the California Environmental Protection Agency*. Smoking and Tobacco Control Monograph 10. National Cancer Institute, Bethesda, MD.

15 Department of Health and Social Security (1988) *Fourth Report on the Independent Scientific Committee on Smoking and Health*. Department of Health and Social Security, London.

16 Smith-Warner SA, Speigelman D, Yaun SS *et al*. (1998) Alcohol and breast cancer in women. *JAMA*. **279**: 535–40.

17 Snyderwine EG (1996) Food derived from heterocyclic amines as etiologic agents in human mammary cancer. *Cancer*. **74**: 1070–7.

18 Cummings JH, Bingham SA, Heaton KW and Eastwood MA (1992) Fecal weight, colon cancer risk and dietary intake of non-starch polysaccharides (dietary fibre). *Gastroenterology*. **103**: 1783–9.

19 Roberts-Thompson IC, Ryan P, Khoo KK, Hart WJ, McMichael AJ and Butler RN (1996) Diet, acetylator phenotype, and risk of colorectal neoplasia. *Lancet*. **347**: 1372–4.

20 Selley S, Donovan J, Faulkner A, Coast J and Gillat D (1997) Diagnosis, management and screening of early localised prostate cancer. *Health Technol Assess*. **1**: 1–72.

21 Lew EA and Garfinkel LL (1979) Variations in mortality by weight among 750 000 men and women. *J Chron Dis*. **32**: 563–76.

22 Martland HS (1931) The occurrence of malignancy in radioactive persons. *Am J Cancer*. **15**: 2435–516.

23 Cardis E and Kaldor J (1989) Radiation and cancer: overview and implications for prevention. In: T Heller, B Davey and L Bailey (eds) *Reducing the Risk of Cancers*. Hodder and Stoughton, London, 51–7.

24 Kennedy CA, Gray AM, Denman AR and Phillips PS (1999) A cost-effectiveness analysis of a residential radon remediation programme in the United Kingdom. *Br J Cancer.* **81**: 1243–7.

25 Ness AR, Frankel SJ, Gunnell D and Davey-Smith G (1999) Are we really dying for a tan? *BMJ.* **319**: 114–16.

26 Elwood JM and Jopson J (1997) Melanoma and sun exposure: an overview of published studies. *Int J Cancer.* **73**: 198–203.

27 Adami J, Frisch M, Yuen J, Glimelius B and Melbye M (1995) Evidence of an association between non-Hodgkin's lymphoma and skin cancer. *BMJ.* **310**: 1491–5.

28 McPherson KM, Steel CM, and Dixon JM (1995) Breast cancer – epidemiology, risk factors and genetics. In: JM Dixon (ed.) *ABC of Breast Diseases*. BMJ Books, London, 18–21.

29 Doll R and Peto R (1981) The causes of cancer: quantitative estimates of avoidable risks of cancer in the United States today. *J Natl Cancer Inst.* **66**: 1191–308.

30 Doll R and Peto R (1985) *Asbestos: effects on health of exposure to asbestos*. Health and Safety Commission, London.

31 Camus M, Siemiatycki J and Meek B (1998) Non-occupational exposure to chrysotile asbestos and the risk of lung cancer. *NEJM.* **338**: 1565–71.

32 Vannio H (1992) Occupational cancer prevention. In: T Heller, L Bailey and S Pattison (eds) *Preventing Cancers*. Open University Press, Buckingham, 78–90.

33 Barbone F, Bovenzi M, Cavelleri F and Stanta G (1995) Air pollution and lung cancer in Trieste, Italy. *Am J Epidemiol.* **141**: 1161–9

34 Katsouyanni K and Pershagen G (1997) Ambient air pollution exposure and cancer. *Cancer Causes Control.* **8**: 284–91.

35 Levi F (1999) Cancer prevention: epidemiology and perspectives. *Euro J Cancer.* **35**: 1912–24.

36 Parkin DM, Pisani P and Ferlay J (1990) Estimates of the worldwide incidence of 25 major cancers in 1990. *Int J Cancer.* **80**: 827–41.

37 Gottlieb S (1999) Papillomavirus DNA in smear test raises risk of cervical cancer. *BMJ.* **319**: 1454.

38 Forman D (1991) *Helicobacter pylori* infection: a novel risk factor in the etiology of gastric cancer. *J Natl Cancer Inst.* **83**: 1702–3.

39 Gallo RC (1998) The enigma of Kaposi's sarcoma. *Science.* **282**: 1837–9.

CHAPTER 6

Calman–Hine and after

Geoff Hall, Peter Selby and Tim Perren

Introduction

In 1995, when an Expert Advisory Group on Cancer (EAGC), expertly led by Sir Kenneth Calman, came up with proposals for reorganisation of cancer care, these suggestions were generally welcomed. However, it was recognised that the recommendations were significantly counter to the prevailing management culture in the NHS at that time. The proposals were to establish, across the country, collaborative networks of care focusing on the needs of patients and their families and providing their care near to home where possible, and in more distant but fully developed and equipped cancer centres when necessary.

At that time the NHS was entering the final phase of an internal market philosophy that did not encourage co-operation between hospitals or joint planning for the movement of patients into the most appropriate location for their care. There was also a long history of reports recommending changes in cancer care and a recognition that many of these reports had not successfully resulted in beneficial change. Therefore the signs were not very encouraging. However, the Calman–Hine proposals have maintained credibility and a degree of implementation has occurred. As we now begin to consider the next phase of the development of cancer services in the NHS Cancer Plan (NCP), it is timely to assess what has been achieved following the Calman–Hine plan, to what degree a platform for future developments has been provided, and to learn from its successes and failures to ensure that the NCP can be more comprehensively successful.

The Calman–Hine proposed structure for cancer services

The principles that govern the development of the Calman–Hine plan have been stated often, but will bear repeating here.

- All patients should have access to a uniformly high quality of care.
- There should be public and professional education to help early recognition of the symptoms of cancer.
- Patients and their families and carers should be given clear information and assistance.
- The development of cancer services should be patient centred and should take into account patients', families' and carers' views.
- The primary care team is a central and continuing element in cancer care.
- Psychosocial aspects of cancer care should be considered.
- Cancer registration and careful monitoring of treatment and outcomes are essential.

The structure proposed was pragmatic and recommended a network of care at three levels:

- *primary care teams*, as the focus of care
- *designated cancer units*, created in district general hospitals, if they had sufficient expertise and facilities to manage common cancers
- *designated cancer centres*, providing a high standard of comprehensive, specialised and multidisciplinary care for most cancers, including rare cases.

This structure was pragmatic because it was achievable within the general framework of medical care within the UK. It was felt to be inadvisable to question the appropriateness of the three tiers of care that currently prevail, but rather to try to develop a plan that could work effectively within that structure. The idea of a network of care was again a pragmatic attempt to put some precision, structure and formality into the referral processes that had operated for many years. However, it was specifically intended that it should not remain a matter of chance or special medical enthusiasm that would determine where and by whom a patient was treated during the acute phase of their management.

One other piece of background information may be relevant here. The Calman–Hine Plan was in a formal sense 'evidence based'. The evidence review that was included in the plan was a powerful influence over its development. Although the evidence was incomplete and imperfect, it provided powerful pointers towards the development of the plan and a powerful defence of the plan when it was criticised, as was inevitably the case, from many quarters. The evidence for site-specialised and multidisciplinary cancer care delivered in sufficient quantity to establish and maintain excellence was quite strong at the time of preparation, and the evidence base has strengthened considerably in the last five years. It was intended that detailed evidence reviews would be necessary for every cancer site, and detailed further work on the guidance that would be appropriate in planning the service would follow site by site in the following years.

This developmental and relatively non-prescriptive approach defined by the Calman–Hine Report had the merit of leaving further work and implementation in the hands of healthcare commissioners, providers and a wide range of healthcare professionals. The absence of a fixed blueprint did allow flexibility. It was probably inevitable, and certainly the case, that this flexibility created a loophole through which those who were too preoccupied with other matters managed to escape. On the other hand, flexibility and the lack of a prescriptive approach strengthened the position of those who were committed to improving cancer services.

Updating the evidence

The evidence base depended on three themes.[1,2]

1   The international comparisons between the UK and comparable European countries that were made by the Eurocare investigators[3,4] showed UK outcomes to be at the lower end of the range in most cancer types, and there was a disturbing consistency about the data. Although the methods of data collection varied and the selection of registered data that could be used had to be limited, there were real grounds for concern following these international comparisons.
2   Within the UK, comparisons of specialised with less specialised medical care gave a consistent picture of survival benefits for patients who were managed in specialised services with the appropriate specialists and the appropriate volumes of work. In no case is there a complete body of data that allows every aspect of specialised care (the specialist, the volume of work, the support team or the available facilities) to be separately and independently evaluated. However, there is quite a strong consensus favouring specialised care for many cancers.[1,2]
3   The processes of care in the UK were seen to be inadequate. It was apparent that there were too few specialists, too few facilities and inadequate expenditure on the necessary tools of the trade for specialists in all aspects of cancer care. In addition, substantially lower expenditure on chemotherapy and a lower uptake of chemotherapy in the UK compared with other Western European countries has been noted.

Although each individual piece of evidence is imperfect, a consistent picture emerges with the evidence suggesting that there are a substantial number of unnecessary deaths from cancer in the UK because of inadequate care. It is difficult to be precise about the scale of the problem because of the lack of precision in the data. However, a few comments can be made. The apparent shortfall in survival compared with other Western European countries is often in excess of 10% at ten years. These figures have to be treated with caution because of the difficulties in interpreting the data collection processes, and in some cases differences of this size are implausible. The data on the impact of specialised care within the UK are perhaps more immediately relevant, since they imply an association with UK care processes. When the many studies looking at different aspects of specialisation in breast cancer were subjected to an overview analysis, the overall difference in survival was 18%. Again this seems large, given that the differences in these patterns of practice probably reflect the impact of care rather than the timing of the diagnosis. Most treatment interventions in breast cancer, such as adjuvant chemotherapy or hormonal therapy, have an impact on survival that is less than 10% at five years. The omission of individual interventions might therefore not be expected to result in a decrease in survival of more than 10%. Where specific comparisons of populations who receive specialised compared with non-specialised care were possible, as in the Glasgow analysis of specialised care in breast cancer,[5] they suggested a 5–10% survival advantage from best available specialised care for breast cancer. Similar analyses for gastrointestinal cancer and ovarian cancer again suggest survival benefits in the range 5–10%.[1]

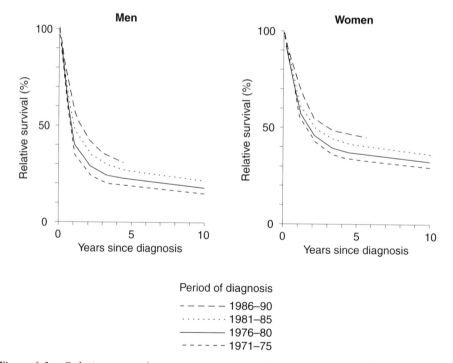

Figure 6.1: Relative survival up to ten years: trends by calendar period of diagnosis during the period 1971–90, for England and Wales.[6]

Given the lack of precision of the data, we would suggest that cautious interpretation is appropriate, but that overall the evidence suggests that the loss of survival at five years is unlikely to be less than 5%, which implies that there are in excess of 10 000 unnecessary deaths from cancer in the UK per annum.

More recent studies of cancer survival trends in England and Wales are more encouraging but also raise some concerns. Since 1971 there has been an increase in the proportion of cancer patients who survive that has been steady and has been observed in many cancer sites.[6] Figure 6.1 shows the survival curves (five years on five years) for men and women in England and Wales. The increase in survival every five years is about 4%. This will vary between different cancer sites and will of course depend on the mix of cases. However the trend is encouraging.

The data on the impact of social deprivation on cancer survival were less encouraging.[6] Figure 6.2 shows a consistent variation in many cancer sites between survival in affluent and deprived communities, and Table 6.1 shows the data in more detail. Explanations for the poor survival rates in deprived communities are likely to be complex, and we should not assume that this is a reflection of inadequate care or poor access to care. Other features of the populations must also be considered, including nutritional status and environmental

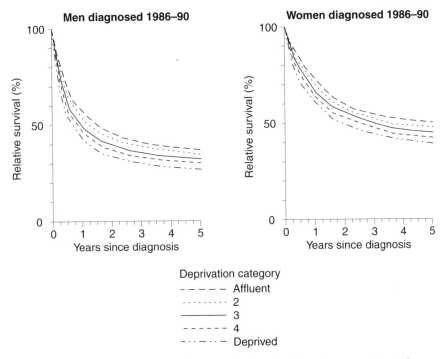

Figure 6.2: Relative survival up to five years, by deprivation category: patients diagnosed during the period 1986–90, for England and Wales.[6]

Table 6.1: Relative survival by deprivation category (all cancers combined, adults diagnosed in England and Wales during 1986–90), and difference (deprivation gap) between most affluent and most deprived categories

	Deprivation category					
	Affluent	2	3	4	Deprived	Deprivation gap
Number of patients	(147 124)	(163 847)	(167 543)	(161 597)	(133 383)	(773 494)
One-year survival (%)	62.6	59.8	57.1	53.3	49.9	−12.7
Five-year survival (%)	43.4	40.8	38.6	35.3	32.3	−11.1

Source: adapted from Coleman *et al.*[6]

exposure. It is noteworthy that the survival rates in the affluent communities in England and Wales are comparable with the best survival rates in other Western European countries when comparisons with the Eurocare studies are made.

The overall explanation for the poor cancer outcomes in the UK is not entirely clear. Different 'interest groups' immediately identified their own special area as being the most important one for remedy. However, it is likely that a number of factors contribute to poor outcomes, including a slow and poorly targeted referral process from the primary sector into secondary care, inadequate facilities and staff which slow down and limit the quality of the diagnostic work-up, and poor resourcing of the secondary and tertiary treatment facilities in both surgical and non-surgical areas.

A full examination of the evidence for these conclusions has now been made for breast cancer, colorectal cancer, lung cancer, gynaecological cancers and upper gastrointestinal cancers and published both with guidance for the development of appropriate services and a summary of the research evidence by the NHS Executive.[7–16]

The initial reaction to the Calman–Hine Report

The service framework proposed in the Calman–Hine document was briskly debated. Criticisms came from several directions. Some felt that the suggestion that cancer centres had to be identified, and that there were some aspects of care that should only be delivered in centres with adequate facilities, specialisation and multidisciplinary teams, might deplete the services available in nearby district hospitals. Others felt that it would not be possible to deliver care of equal specialisation or with equal technical resources in district hospitals at all. These conflicting views have been resolved into the recognition that there is a case for substantial change. The development of evidence-based guidelines for each cancer has vastly improved the quality of the debate, and a broad consensus about the need to change and the nature of the recommendations has emerged. The proposals are now supported in principle by healthcare professionals, health service managers and the Department of Health.[17]

Changes in the first five years

Each English region and Scotland, Wales and Northern Ireland took rather different approaches to the implementation of the Calman–Hine recommendations. Some were vigorous, developing regionwide working parties and reviewing cancer services in cancer centres and cancer units with review visits. Specific programmes for service development were proposed with revisiting required. In some regions very detailed standards for these exercises were developed. This has resulted in change, although it remains patchy. There is evidence of a greater degree of specialisation and multidisciplinary working for common cancers in district hospitals. For instance, in the Northern and Yorkshire region, the proportion of patients with breast cancer who are seen by a specialist surgeon (defined as one who sees more than 50 patients with breast cancer each year) is now well above 50% for the first time. There have been cancer centres identified at the heart of 34 cancer networks in England and in Wales. However, the designation of a cancer centre is not always consistent with that recommended in the original Calman–Hine Report, and many of them are considerably smaller than the optimal size.

The Calman–Hine Report recommended that substantial growth was necessary in the provision of non-surgical oncology support to district hospitals. A minimum of five sessions per cancer unit was recommended. In a recent analysis, Haward and Amir surveyed the provision of non-surgical oncology care in cancer units across England and Wales, and showed that there has been a substantial increase (from 20% to 60%) in the proportion of responding units that meet the minimum standard.[18]

Issues, problems and pitfalls

In general, implementation remains far from complete and the processes for its evaluation are still inconsistent across the countries of the UK.[19] In particular:

- there has been considerably less progress in involving the primary care community in the implementation of the Calman–Hine recommendations than is necessary or desirable
- the provision of care in cancer units and cancer centres has become more multidisciplinary and specialised, but this process is incomplete
- although the strengthening of services for common cancers in district hospitals is advanced, reconfiguration of services following guidance for cancers of intermediate frequency is only just beginning. The reconfigurations that are required as recommended by, for instance, the Gynaecological Cancer Guidance are substantial and potentially expensive
- until recently, no adequate or relevant resource increase was available
- the new service patterns and the identified unmet need in cancer care put tremendous pressure on training and manpower
- data collection and audit and monitoring outcomes are still patchy and inadequate.

Cancer networks

Both the Calman–Hine Report and the NHS Cancer Plan[20] emphasise the importance of establishing functional networks of primary, secondary and tertiary care to deliver cancer services. Networks combine and require integrated working between a variety of trusts which are commonly linked through several health authorities and large numbers of primary care trusts. The concept of a cancer network is really a novel and systematic attempt to harmonise practice, develop the organisation of service delivery and improve the experience of patients. Networks are an important means of developing and modernising cancer services on a rational and integrated basis, and it is expected that cancer networks will ultimately develop to govern the flow of patients by the adoption of national guidance and local policies. This approach has considerable merit and support, but its supporters often emphasise very different aspects of cancer networks. On the one hand, many professional oncologists and managers regard networks as vehicles for change, with the potential for radical reconfiguration of services within the network in order to implement the guidance for cancers of intermediate frequency. On the other hand, the availability of a 'network' may be regarded by some as allowing the status quo to continue with everyone included but no real change. A great deal of work is therefore necessary to substantiate and strengthen the function of cancer networks. In our experience, the following conditions are necessary for their success:

- clear and precise aims, structures and responsibilities
- an agreed remit that is nationally consistent

- the adoption and generation of guidance/guidelines, preferably nationally
- data collection with 'no hiding places'
- visit-based 'accreditation' of services
- connection to operational NHS management at the highest level (CEOs)
- connection to resources at network level through joint commissioning
- winning professional 'hearts and minds' by explanation and persuasion
- resources and time for key staff to work on network development.

The NHS Cancer Plan

The NHS Cancer Plan, which was published in September 2000, describes a five year plan for cancer services development. The Plan builds on the experience with the Calman–Hine Report to set out a comprehensive national cancer programme that extends planning beyond service development, which was the principal focus of the Calman–Hine recommendations, to include prevention with a particular emphasis on the reduction of smoking in adults. This broader remit has been widely welcomed among the cancer-related professions in England.

Many of the goals of the Calman–Hine Report are retained, but the NHS Cancer Plan has specificity and resource allocations that should greatly enhance the efforts to save lives and improve the quality of life of patients with cancer.

It is associated with new funding rising to £570 million per year for cancer services by 2003/2004. By 2006 there are plans to have 1000 extra cancer specialists, with more radiographers, more nurses and targeted action to develop the workforce with funding for equipment and facilities also identified. A detailed review of the NHS Cancer Plan is beyond the remit of this chapter, and the reader is referred to the Plan itself and its useful Executive Summary.[20]

The Cancer Plan allows for the following:

- new national and local targets to reduce smoking in disadvantaged groups
- new local alliances for action on smoking
- support in primary care to help people to quit smoking
- £2.5 million for research into smoking cessation
- national five-a-day programme to increase fruit and vegetable consumption
- national School Fruit Scheme
- raising public awareness

The achievement of a reduction in smoking has the greatest potential for reducing cancer deaths and could, if successful, lead to as much as a 10% reduction in cancer death rates within 10 years.

Other risk factors, such as obesity, physical inactivity, alcohol, excessive sun exposure and radiation exposure, are also tackled, and work to promote an improved diet is planned and resourced.

The following screening improvements are proposed:

- routine breast screening to be extended up to the age of 70 years and available on request to women over the age of 70 years
- improved breast screening techniques to increase detection rates
- improved cervical screening techniques
- colorectal screening pilots
- the NHS Prostate Cancer Programme
- the promotion of a better understanding of screening.

The ideal test for screening for colorectal cancer has yet to be established, although the majority of large randomised trials support the utility of faecal occult blood testing.[21] The potential for effective approaches to screening for prostate cancer, ovarian cancer and lung cancer is still being evaluated, and as yet there is no definite evidence that lives will be saved by their introduction in the UK.

Primary care

The NHS Cancer Plan confirms and extends the recommendations of the Calman–Hine Report in the area of primary care oncology. Specific proposals are as follows:

- a central role for primary care in new cancer networks
- £3 million in partnership with Macmillan for a lead cancer clinician in every primary care trust
- £2 million for palliative care training for district nurses
- a new primary care clinical dataset for cancer patients.

Such proposals are necessary if we are to see improvements in care and the reduction in time to referral that is essential to improve survival.

For the development of secondary and tertiary cancer services, the work started by the Calman–Hine Report and the National Cancer Guidance exercises will be adopted by the National Institute for Clinical Excellence with an active programme of guidance to be issued until mid-2003, and a new approach to the appraisal of cancer drugs and their availability. Although the success of this approach has yet to be demonstrated, the specificity of the consideration of the need for cancer drugs is widely welcomed. Specific allocations for palliative care

Table 6.2: Anticipated consultant numbers

Medical (England only)	1999	2003–04	2005–06	Increase (1999–2006)	Increase (%) 1999–2006
Histopathologists	836	913	968	+132	16
Radiologists	1507	1840	1767	+260	17
Clinical oncologists	305	420	453	+148	49
Medical oncologists	110	192	265	+155	141
Haematologists	510	639	659	+149	29
Palliative care physicians	94	164	221	+127	135
Total	3362	4169	4333	+971	29

Source: Department of Health.[20]

resources, with £50 million extra for hospices and specialist palliative care services, may well allow the implementation of developments in this area.

Workforce

The NHS Cancer Plan sets out for the first time the agenda for increasing the numbers of available medical consultants whose contributions to cancer care are specific (*see* Table 6.2). It is important to emphasise that many other medical specialties contribute to the care of cancer patients, and developments in surgery and medicine, gynaecology and many other fields will also be important in the coming years. Diagnostic and therapeutic radiographers and medical physicists play a critical role, with increases to the year 2006 planned of 4%, 16% and 12%, respectively. The central role of cancer nurses in providing for the needs of cancer patients is well recognised both on the ward, as nurse specialists and in the delivery of treatments (including chemotherapy) and, of course, in palliative care in hospices and hospitals as well as in the community.

The role of cancer research in developing the cancer service

A great deal of knowledge has been generated by basic and clinical cancer research in recent years, and this has already led to significant improvements in many aspects of cancer prevention and treatment. The rate of accumulation of new knowledge is now very rapid, and its potential for translation into the clinical area is also great. For example, new ideas in molecular pathology and in pharmacology and immunology will probably change the shape of cancer diagnosis and treatment in the next ten years. This is clearly significant for the NHS in a host of different ways. The shape of service delivery will change, and the facilities that are necessary for it will also change. On the one hand, the requirements for centralisation of services may increase as a result of innovations involving high technology and large amounts of equipment. On the other hand, in some areas the need for central referral may decrease as treatments and management strategies can be safely delivered in cancer units.

This need for new knowledge and the interpretation of knowledge from basic sciences in itself makes a strong case for a major commitment to research within cancer services in the NHS. The NHS cannot rely on the voluntary sector or pharmaceutical industry to provide its evidence base.

In addition to the need to accumulate and evaluate new knowledge and translate it into 'new medicine', there is an additional case for a portfolio of research within our cancer services. The evidence consistently suggests that patients who are managed within clinical trials or who are managed in institutions that are committed to clinical trials have better outcomes.[22,23] These benefits for patients as a result of the trials activity within their institution relate to the quality of care that is dictated by trials protocols and to the commitment to protocol-based care that is a feature of teams which are conducting clinical trials. Research clinicians are committed to the high standards of care that follow from their trials, as well as to advancing medical knowledge.[24] Thus participation in trials is a good indicator of high-quality care. Slevin and colleagues have shown that the vast majority of patients support clinical trials and understand that research is associated with excellent specialised treatment.[25] Patients and clinical investigators are committed to the clinical trials environment as a vehicle for excellent treatment.[26,27]

In order to address these issues, a cancer working party on priorities in NHS research and development, identified the need for infrastructure to support clinical research, in both randomised prospective trials and other well-designed studies, in their report to the NHS R&D Strategic Priority Review in 1998.[28] Building on this, NHS Research and Development has developed a proposal for a National Cancer Research Network that will provide the infrastructure for such clinical research, and which will work with the other cancer research funders to enhance both the quality and breadth of, and participation in, the clinical trials conducted within the cancer networks. Funding for this activity will increase to £20 million per annum in the next few years, and should not only result in the accrual of new knowledge but also make a contribution to the improvement in cancer care standards.

The reorganisation of cancer services: a worked example

The concept of a local cancer hospital (either a cancer unit or a cancer centre) providing cancer care for local patients with common cancers (i.e. lung, breast and colorectal cancers) is broadly accepted and well provided within the current model of cancer service provision. More contentious is the provision of cancer care for patients with less common cancers at cancer centres where the degree of specialisation required to achieve clinical excellence is more likely to be ensured.

Gynaecological cancer services within the Yorkshire Cancer Network

Gynaecological cancers are considerably less frequent than the three common cancers. A cancer unit that serves 250 000 people is likely to see approximately one new case of ovarian cancer per fortnight and less than one new case of endometrial cancer per fortnight. They therefore represent cancers of intermediate frequency which exemplify the proposed plan for centralised cancer care. A proposal for the organisation of such services was central to the *Guidance for Commissioning Cancer Services Report on Gynaecological Cancers* published by the NHS Executive in 1999. The key recommendations of this report were as follows:

- diagnostic and assessment units to be established in cancer units
- specialist multiprofessional gynaecological oncology teams based in cancer centres to be responsible for the management of all patients with ovarian cancer and most patients with other gynaecological malignancies
- defined local policies to be agreed between the cancer centre and its associated cancer units on the management of women with advanced or progressive disease
- efficient communication between all elements of the cancer network, including regional audit of service delivery.

The Yorkshire Cancer Network has decided to embrace these guidelines, and is reconfiguring gynaecological cancer services to incorporate the changes that are required. These changes will be made in two phases. The first phase centralised gynaecological cancer services within Leeds in November 2001, leading to network-wide centralisation by 2003. This means that, annually,

Table 6.3: Annual referrals within the Yorkshire Cancer Network to the Leeds Cancer Centre

Site of cancer	Current cancer centre referrals	Potential cancer centre referrals	Cases diagnosed in Yorkshire Region
Ovary	97	272	359
Cervix	76	205	293
Uterus	63	176	248
Total	236	653	889

the management of more than 650 cases (*see* Table 6.3) of gynaecological cancer patients will be co-ordinated at the Leeds Cancer Centre within Improving Outcomes in Cancer Guidance.

This will require considerable service reorganisation. The gynaecological cancer surgery that is currently performed at two centres within Leeds and at least eight other hospitals across the region will be performed within a single centre (St James's University Hospital, Leeds). The increased number of patients undergoing surgery within the centre will require an increase in the number of consultant gynaecological surgical oncologists, with a corresponding increase in the number of beds, operating time and out-patient consultation space available to the surgical team. The centralisation will significantly increase the workload of the other related specialties, such as pathology and radiology. An increase in consultant numbers for these specialties has also been planned and has in part already been implemented to support the proposed changes.

The reconfiguration of non-surgical gynaecological oncology services within the Yorkshire Cancer Network has required less radical changes. Radiotherapy will continue to be delivered at a single centre (currently Cookridge Hospital), although it is planned to move this service to the St James's site by 2006–07. Chemotherapy is currently administered at a number of district general hospitals within the network. At those hospitals with resident medical oncologists, where patients have 24-hour access to specialist support, patients will continue to be offered chemotherapy at their local cancer unit. However, this chemotherapy will only be given from within a portfolio of regimens and clinical trials that are agreed regionally. Treatment with high-dose chemotherapy, phase I trials and trials of novel biological agents will be run centrally, with patients generally receiving such treatment at the centre (i.e. St James's University Hospital, Leeds). An essential part of the decision to allow chemotherapy to be administered at many hospitals within the Leeds Cancer Network will be the use of IT strategies to enable network-wide review of all treatments, toxicities and outcomes.

Central to the successful implementation of this network-wide reconfiguration is the weekly multi-disciplinary team (MDT) meeting at which all patients who have been diagnosed with gynaecological cancer within the region are discussed. Surgical and non-surgical oncologists with a specialist interest in the management of patients with gynaecological cancer at cancer units affiliated to the Leeds Cancer Centre are able to bring cases for discussion at this meeting. This ensures that the combined expertise of the regional team is available to every patient, in order to make certain that the very highest standards of care are uniformly available to all patients.

The process of investigation, diagnosis and subsequent treatment of patients with gynaecological cancer has therefore been modified within the Yorkshire Cancer Network to accommodate the essential recommendations of the *Guidance for Commissioning Cancer Services Report on Gynaecological Cancers* published by the NHS Executive in 1999 (i.e. local diagnosis, regional review of management and treatment within protocols agreed across the network). The framework defined within this guidance document has been key to its successful implementation, and has facilitated the acceptance of significant change by many professionals within the region. However, the successful implementation of the plans will rely on the outstanding commitment and goodwill of staff towards beneficial change when they know that it is both possible and achievable.

It is hoped that such a reconfiguration will facilitate the vision of cancer care defined by both the Calman–Hine Report and the more recent NHS Improving Outcomes guidelines. The increase in patient numbers will lead to more extensive experience for medical professionals as well as enhanced research opportunities, both of which should improve the quality of care delivered – a level of care to which all patients across the network will have equal access.

Conclusions

It is now recognised that there has been a pressing need for improvements in cancer services, and that these improvements can result in thousands of lives being saved. The process is complex, but there is now a great deal of consensus about the principles that should be followed and the details of their implementation. Progress has been slow and the work to date has been under-resourced, but nevertheless there have been real achievements. Matters are now better planned and resourced under the NHS Cancer Plan, and it is reasonable to anticipate a period of steady and substantial progress. There may be limitations on the pace of progress arising from the limited availability of skilled staff and the many other pressures and challenges which operate within health services. However, there is a real opportunity to further strengthen and improve cancer services, to broaden the base of that improvement to include prevention, and to adopt a fresh approach to the implementation of the ideas of the Calman–Hine plan and the recommendations that have been proposed since then.

References

1 Selby P, Gillis C and Haward R (1996) Benefits from specialised cancer care. *Lancet.* **348**: 313–18.

2 Hillner BE, Smith TJ and Desch CE (2000) Hospital and physician volume or specialization and outcomes in cancer treatment: importance in quality of cancer care. *J Clin Oncol.* **18**: 2327–40.

3 Berrino F, Sant M, Verdecchia A *et al.* (eds) (1995) *Survival of Cancer Patients in Europe: the EUROCARE Study.* IARC Scientific Publications No 132. International Agency for Research on Cancer, Lyon.

4 Berrino F, Capocaccia J, Estève G *et al.* (eds) (1999) *Survival of Cancer Patients in Europe: the EUROCARE-2 Study.* IARC Scientific Publications No 151. International Agency for Research on Cancer, Lyon.

5 Gillis CR and Hole DJ (1996) Survival outcome of care by specialist surgeons in breast cancer: a study of 3786 patients in the west of Scotland. *BMJ.* **312**: 145–8.

6 Coleman MP, Babb P, Damiecki P *et al.* (eds) (1999) *Cancer Survival Trends in England and Wales 1971–1995: deprivation and NHS region.* The Stationery Office, London.

7 NHS Executive (1996) *Improving Outcomes in Breast Cancer: the manual.* NHS Executive, Leeds.

8 NHS Executive (1996) *Improving Outcomes in Breast Cancer: the research evidence.* NHS Executive, Leeds.

9 NHS Executive (1997) *Improving Outcomes in Colorectal Cancer: the manual.* NHS Executive, Leeds.

10 NHS Executive (1997) *Improving Outcomes in Colorectal Cancer: the research evidence.* NHS Executive, Leeds.

11 NHS Executive (1998) *Improving Outcomes in Lung Cancer: the manual.* NHS Executive, Leeds.

12 NHS Executive (1998) *Improving Outcomes in Lung Cancer: the research evidence.* NHS Executive, Leeds.

13 NHS Executive (1999) *Improving Outcomes in Gynaecological Cancer: the manual.* NHS Executive, Leeds.

14 NHS Executive (1999) *Improving Outcomes in Gynaecological Cancer: the research evidence.* NHS Executive, Leeds.

15 NHS Executive (2000) *Improving Outcomes in Upper Gastrointestinal Cancer: the manual.* NHS Executive, Leeds.

16 NHS Executive (2000) *Improving Outcomes in Upper Gastrointestinal Cancer: the research evidence.* NHS Executive, Leeds.

17 Department of Health (1998) *A First-Class Service. Quality in the new NHS – consultation document.* The Stationery Office, London.

18 Haward RA and Amir Z (2000) Progress in establishing non-surgical oncology within English cancer units. *Br J Cancer.* **83**: 284–6.

19 Selby P and Haward R (1998) Calman proposals for cancer: where are they going? *Hosp Med.* **59**: 836–7.

20 Department of Health (2000) *The NHS Cancer Plan.* Department of Health, London.

21 Mandel JS, Church TR, Bond JH *et al.* (2000) The effect of fecal occult-blood screening on the incidence of colorectal cancer. *NEJM.* **343**: 1603–7.

22 Karjalainen S and Palva I (1989) Do treatment protocols improve end results? A study of survival of patients with multiple myeloma in Finland. *BMJ.* **299**: 1069–72.

23 Stiller CA (1989) Survival of patients with cancer: those included in trials do better. *BMJ.* **299**: 1058–9.

24 Taylor KM (1992) Physician participation in a randomised clinical trial for ocular melanoma. *Ann Ophthalmol.* **24**: 337–44.

25 Slevin M, Mossman J, Bowling A *et al.* (1995) Volunteers or victims: patients' views of randomised cancer clinical trials. *Br J Cancer.* **71**: 1270–74.

26 Cockburn J, Redman S and Kricker A (1998) Should women take part in clinical trials in breast cancer? Issues and some solutions. *J Clin Oncol.* **16**: 354–62.

27 Moore O (1996) *PWA: looking AIDS in the face.* Picador, London.

28 Cancer Topic Working Party (1998) *Report to NHS Research and Development Strategic Priority Review.* Cancer Topic Working Party, London.

CHAPTER 7

Commissioning cancer services

Robert Haward, Ian Manifold and John Wilkinson

Commissioning in the NHS: a general introduction

Commissioning is a relatively recent concept which has crept into common parlance in the NHS in England and Wales over recent years. Its origin and growing usage can be traced back to the NHS reforms[1] of the late 1980s, which heralded the introduction of the internal market into the NHS. These launched the internal market, creating NHS trusts and separating the providing functions of healthcare organisations from what was then referred to as the purchaser role. Over subsequent years the language of the internal market was gradually moderated. In the early days of the internal market, the terms 'contracting', 'purchasing' and 'commissioning' were used almost interchangeably, but gradually the term 'purchasing' gave way to a more broadly acceptable function – that of 'commissioning'. Commissioning was defined by Sheaff and Peel[2] as 'the use of purchasing power to influence what health care providers have available, to develop and shape the internal market itself, and in these ways to influence what direction both the health systems as a whole and technologies develop in. This would include encouraging new providers to enter the internal market (or old ones to leave)'. The process of commissioning is summarised in Box 7.1. Commissioning replaced the market model, characterised by its rejection of formal planning systems, with new processes that shared many features with what was formerly regarded in the NHS as strategic and operational planning.

However, during the late 1980s and most of the 1990s the market approach dominated the way in which health services were provided. The market was

---

Box 7.1:   Commissioning: the cycle of managerial activities

1   Articulate purchaser's commissioning objectives.
2   Establish facts about resident population's health status.
3   Establish facts about existing service provision, use and demand.
4   Articulate purchaser's health targets.
5   Establish variances between targets, actual health status, service provision, service use and unmet demand. Establish main consequences of these variances.
6   Decide on possible interventions.
7   Service specification: service mix, quantities, cost, quality.
8   Determine criteria for awarding service contract.
9   Produce action list with costed options of current and alternative providers.
10   Select provider(s).
11   Negotiate with selected provider(s).
12   Let service contract.
13   Monitor provider compliance with contract.
14   Payment, remedy or sanctions.
15   Review impact on health status.

Source: Best Practice in Health Care Commissioning.[2]

---

particularly detrimental to co-ordinated care across organisational boundaries, as it generated competition between hospitals, thereby discouraging collaboration. Investment in major developments in specialised and centralised services, normally located in tertiary centres, was much more difficult to achieve. For cancer services there were unfortunate consequences. Investment in high-cost equipment such as linear accelerators – used in much of cancer treatment and with capital costs in excess of £1 million – became much less co-ordinated for both replacement and new machines. Healthcare purchasers tended to concentrate their efforts and resources on their local services. The decline in some specialised facilities in major centres was further exacerbated by the radical diminution of the regional role in strategic planning. This was brought about by the merger (from 14 down to 8) and then abolition[3] of regional health authorities (RHAs) between 1994 and 1996, with radical staff reductions. RHAs had until then exercised formal responsibilities for the planning and commissioning of specialist services, which had included some cancer services. They were replaced by regional offices of the NHS Executive. These bodies were initially required to devolve responsibility for much of their previous service and capital planning activities to health authorities, until a further change in government policy[4] sought to re-establish some of these roles, although within a different framework, during 1998 and 1999. Regional offices were asked to pay particular attention to commissioning of cancer services.[5]

There were initially two types of purchasers/commissioners, namely GP fundholders and health authorities. Fundholders were responsible for purchasing/commissioning a limited range of services, mainly low-cost elective services, from local NHS trusts. Health authorities were responsible for commissioning more complex services. In a limited number of places GP total funds were set up, usually covering populations of over 50 000, which were responsible for commissioning almost all services to meet the needs of their patients.

There was always a gap between the theory and practice of commissioning. In reality, much commissioning was preoccupied with the mechanics of the process, such as the agreeing of contracts – often a crude process of transferring money between health authorities and trusts – leading to very limited improvements or changes in services. A number of improvements in local services were claimed by GP fundholders.[6] These included the employment of a wider range of staff within the practice, negotiating shorter waiting times for hospital services, and improved use of prescribing budgets. There was more serious concern[7] about differential access to hospital appointments and to elective surgery for the patients of GP fundholders. This led to public and political concern as to whether or not this had resulted in a 'two-tier health service'. It was also described pejoratively as 'a postcode lottery'.

Following the UK election of the Labour Government in 1997, many of the obvious features of the internal market were swept away. However, the new Labour administration did retain the split between health organisations with responsibilities for commissioning services and those that provided them. The 'two-tier health service' issue was addressed directly by the abolition of GP fundholding. However, the involvement of primary care in service commissioning was strengthened and made comprehensive. Instead of a random mix of individual fundholding and non-fundholding practices, all primary care activities were brought together, with the creation of geographically distinct primary care groups (PCGs). These groups of practices typically had patient populations of between 50 000 and 150 000, and included all practices within that particular area. Many were also coterminous with local authority boundaries. In December 1999, the Department of Health in England issued further guidance on the development of primary care groups and the steps required for change to primary care trusts.[8]

In England, 17 primary care trusts (PCTs) became operational on 1 April 2000. A further 23 PCTs became operational on 1 October 2000. The number of PCTs rose to over 160 in April 2001 and this model became comprehensive in England a year later. Arrangements in Scotland, Wales and Northern Ireland are different,[9] and are summarised in Box 7.2.

Box 7.2: Differences in NHS primary care organisations in Wales, Scotland and Northern Ireland

Wales
- No primary healthcare trusts.
- A total of 22 local health groups as health authority subcommittees.
- Role for Welsh Assembly.

Scotland
- Only two types of trust – acute hospital and primary care.
- Local healthcare co-operatives.
- Health boards have enhanced powers.
- Local trust chairs are non-executive directors on health boards.

Northern Ireland
- Fundholding continued until April 2001.
- Range of models under discussion.
- Final decision depends on National Assembly.

The beginnings of cancer commissioning

The widespread service problems resulting from the excessively local focus of much purchasing and commissioning led to a growth of interest in finding ways to address the problems of specialised services. Such interests extended far beyond cancer care. However, with regard to cancer services this was given real urgency as a consequence of the publication in 1995 of a major new cancer policy in England and Wales, closely followed by equivalent initiatives in the other home countries. The report,[10] entitled *A Policy Framework for Commissioning Cancer Services*, was widely known as the Calman–Hine Report after the two Chief Medical Officers of England and Wales who set up this hugely influential initiative. The report was widely welcomed in the cancer community, and appeared to strike a positive chord with patients' groups as well as the clinical professions. It required both commissioners and providers to implement substantial changes in their approach to and management of cancer services, and it caused the NHS to address serious underlying problems both at the clinical practice level and in the wider organisation of cancer care.

Initially, collaborative commissioning for cancer services evolved through loose arrangements between neighbouring health authorities to work together in the commissioning of selected aspects (usually the more specialist cancer services), and to deal with major problems of under-investment. As greater attention began to be given to cancer services, more of the consequences of past under-investment began to emerge. Some of these were particularly apparent in the larger centres. A later Department of Health initiative (1998) re-established formal responsibilities[4] at regional and commissioner level for specialist commissioning. As a result, regional offices in England have each developed explicit arrangements for commissioning specialist services, including a number of cancer services. Responsibility for the commissioning of services for some very rare cancers, such as choriocarcinoma, was always undertaken on a national basis.

Cancer screening services also experienced problems during the 1990s. Most of these arose because of specific incidents within hospital trusts. Although health authorities were responsible for commissioning screening services, few of the problems of screening services were identified through commissioning processes. They normally either presented because problems became apparent through the unsatisfactory experiences of particular patients, or they followed established quality checks within the screening services themselves. Ultimately because of an accumulation of concerns, the Government was recommended (and subsequently agreed) to extend the remit of the breast cancer screening services quality assurance programme to cover cervical screening.[11] Quality assurance directors were appointed in all of the NHS regions in England, although responsibility for commissioning screening services remained with health authorities. An established national screening committee, whose role is considered in Chapter 4, takes decisions about the introduction of all new national screening programmes.

Cancer policy and its implementation

Although the Department of Health in England had longstanding interests in radiotherapy service provision, it did not articulate a policy for cancer until the Bagshawe Report[12] on acute services in cancer was published in 1984. However, this report of a working group had no impact and was not followed through in any way. The Calman–Hine Report[10] published in 1995 was thus the first serious government policy on cancer, and had significant influence. It addressed the provision of all aspects of cancer care. The later NHS Cancer Plan,[13] published in 2000, was more comprehensive – a true cancer control policy. It retained the main recommendations of the Calman–Hine Report, but extended the scope of the policy by introducing additional themes over and above service delivery, such as prevention and screening. It also began to address how changes were to be implemented, particularly manpower planning, which was not covered by the Calman–Hine Report. The plan also

had the benefit of clearly identified extra resources, rising in three annual incre-
ments to £570 million by the year 2003.

As a policy framework, the Calman–Hine Report set out a clear strategy for
the organisation and delivery of services from primary care to cancer centres.
Although it had a number of valuable features, the most important aspect was
its ambition. It sought to achieve a consistent high quality of service available to
the whole population. This was in sharp contrast to the historical background,
with abundant evidence[14–16] showing variability from place to place in the processes and outcomes of care, mounting evidence of patient concern, and public
and political dissatisfaction with the contrast between the care available in different places.

There were two main strands to the policy recommendations. The first was
the adoption within the hospital sector of a specialist service model,[17–19]
which had the following features.

- All patients would have access to relevant specialists.
- Clinical disciplines that were regularly involved in the management of
  cancer patients would be specialists in their respective fields.
- All of the professions and disciplines necessary for managing a particular
  tumour type would be drawn together in a multiprofessional, multidisciplinary team (MDT) to deliver services.
- Patient pathways from primary care to specialist teams in local hospitals
  and, where necessary, in tertiary centres would be made explicit, agreed by
  those involved, and backed by sound interprofessional communications.
- Thus hospital specialists working outside MDTs would not become involved
  in the ongoing management of cancer patients, other than as emergencies.

The second major strand of policy was structural.

- It introduced the new concept of the cancer unit – that is, the secondary care
  organisation for cancer services.
- It described for the first time within a UK context the nature and roles of
  cancer centres.
- It described the respective roles of those involved in cancer care – in primary
  care, local hospital services and specialist hospital services – introducing the
  idea of cancer networks, although the nature of these networks was not
  defined in detail.
- It emphasised the fact that local changes were to be underpinned by audit
  and involvement in research.

Although the basic principles and main recommendations were well expressed,
the Calman–Hine Report did not describe how services for individual cancers
might best be configured and how the clinical care of specific groups of patients

might be organised and delivered. The resolution of this issue is dealt with below in the section on the nature and role of cancer guidance (*see* page 104). Responsibility for the implementation of the Calman–Hine recommendations was largely devolved to the eight regional offices in England, and was pursued separately on a national basis in Wales, Scotland and Northern Ireland. As a result, implementation was inconsistent, and the processes for bringing about the necessary changes varied in style, rigour and effectiveness across the UK.

The Calman–Hine vision was of a breakdown of the traditional, patient-unfriendly, vertical divisions of the NHS into a two-level, horizontal structure consisting of centres and units. Centres were effectively defined as functional collections of services, which together provided all secondary care to their immediate population and most of the tertiary care for the same and also a larger population, which served as the referral source for the centre. Units served sections of the larger catchment area outside the centre and provided all of the secondary services, referring tertiary services to the centre to which they related. These structural features of Calman–Hine led to an initial preoccupation with identifying the potential cancer units[20] and cancer centres in each part of the country. In some regions these issues were addressed through processes designed for this task, involving peer review visits to assess candidate hospitals based on detailed proposals. An example[21] is the description of the process in the Northern and Yorkshire region. The early preoccupation with hospital designation was understandable, as these are key structural components within the Calman–Hine system. The initial clinical focus was on arrangements to establish multidisciplinary teams for the three common cancers (breast, colorectal and lung cancer). This often required local developments to ensure that the required posts were in place, and the adjustment of clinical responsibilities between existing clinicians. Specific enhancements were frequently necessary for diagnostic services and non-surgical oncology. The latter have often resulted in greater availability of local chemotherapy services with an expansion in the numbers of non-surgical oncology sessions[22] in cancer units.

Although individual health authorities and GP commissioning organisations were usually active in the commissioning of unit-based cancer services, the commissioning of cancer centre services was a different matter. It was not simply the responsibility of the health authority in which it was based, but it also required effective collaboration between commissioners, the mechanisms for which were largely absent. Improving the linkage between primary care and hospital services, and between all of the hospitals relating to each cancer centre was, if anything, a greater challenge. The NHS reforms of 1989 had reinforced competitive attitudes between hospitals, although a longer historical perspective suggests that collaboration between hospitals was never particularly well developed, apart from that induced by the former regional health authorities through their clinical networks, though there were honourable exceptions, such as paediatric oncology.

The publication of the NHS Cancer Plan[13] made a particular feature of the role of cancer networks. These networks were intended to be at the heart of implementation and local decision making. Explicitly the Cancer Plan set out the expectation that health service commissioners (health authorities, primary care groups and trusts) and providers (including those in primary and community care as well as hospital trusts) would work together within these cancer networks. Where relevant, both the voluntary sector and local authorities would need to be drawn in. These networks were expected to develop strategic plans, implement them together, and monitor the processes of care through clinical governance. Regional offices in England were expected to oversee and co-ordinate the work of cancer networks.

Cancer networks were expected to increase the involvement of managers. In many locations cancer networks had been predominantly clinical, with little support from or involvement of traditional management structures. The expectation that chief executives would be closely involved in cancer networks, as well as their lead clinicians, was new. The government announced its intention (in paragraph 11.17 of the Cancer Plan) to pilot radical new forms of clinically led care, and it aimed to set up a small number of pilots in cancer networks to assess the feasibility of commissioning all cancer services at network level.

Implementing change: the importance of cancer networks

Although the original concept of the cancer network was straightforward at a superficial level, the practicalities were uncertain. So, too, was the extent of the commitment of clinicians and managers in different institutions to work together to put new arrangements in place. Such changes might alter patient flows, with increased clinical responsibilities for some hospitals and reduced clinical responsibilities for others. This was a demanding requirement for a new and relatively untested organisational concept, particularly as trust managers as distinct from their clinicians had been relatively slow to become involved. Although networks began to emerge in most parts of the country between the publication of the Calman–Hine Report and the NHS Cancer Plan, the pace of their development has been uneven and often slow.

The current reality may differ from that suggested by Calman–Hine, and elaborated upon in the NHS Cancer Plan, in the following ways.

- Centres and units have largely been designated as such across the country according to a variety of criteria, resulting in entities which have a varying (and sometimes distant) resemblance to the Calman–Hine model and an uncertain ability to deliver the latter's vision of equal access to uniformly high-quality service.

- The title 'cancer network' has been given to a variety of arrangements, again with an uncertain ability to deliver the vision. In some regions there is geographical overlapping of effective catchment populations, and there can be complex historical referral patterns which may blur the distinctiveness and separation between centres and units.
- There has been even less co-ordination between commissioners than between providers, with a relative failure to implement collaborative arrangements that mirror those being developed for provider networks.

Part of the difficulty was a high degree of uncertainty as to how decisions made within these networks could be carried through to action by all of the component organisations. There were obvious difficulties in generating a coherence of approach to implementing agreed actions unless both health authorities and trusts could find innovative ways of working together effectively. To achieve this required some 'pooling of sovereignty' to manage resources (money and manpower) for agreed common goals for which each organisation still remained individually responsible and accountable. A number of the preconditions for networks to become successful have recently emerged. These factors combined to create a genuine window of opportunity to get things right.

- The accelerating programme of evidence-based national authoritative guidance on the management of specific cancer types (Clinical Outcomes Group and now NICE) has begun explicitly to recommend the distribution of services for particular cancer types and types of treatment between secondary and tertiary levels of service. This needs a real and effective network to allow its successful implementation.

  The recommendations of the National Cancer Guidance addressed the issues of service configuration – who should do what and where. Without such a star to steer by it was too much to expect major issues of this sort to be resolved by local clinicians and managers with inevitable vested interests.

- The Cancer Plan announced a three-year programme of investment in cancer on a greater scale than ever before, and there is sympathy with the view that cancer networks should have a real say in the distribution of these funds.

  This approach was given an early trial by the successive allocation of relatively modest sums of £10 million for implementation of each of the breast, lung and colorectal (and £9 million for gynaecological) cancer guidance. This was imaginatively handled in some parts of the country and stimulated collaboration within the networks involving all of the organisations

*concerned. It led directly to the beginnings of collaboration between com-
missioners in many networks. The NHS Cancer Plan clearly took this
much further, and further guidance is to be funded from the main allocation
for cancer service development as part of the overall plan.*

- There is to be national appraisal of cancer services against a set of national standards,[23] which will provide an opportunity to define networks and their relationship to commissioners, thereby shaping cancer commissioning itself. This will be a network rather than institutionally focused peer review of services.

  *Although not all parts of the country initially employed external peer
  review to assess progress in implementing Calman–Hine, many did so,
  often with enthusiasm. In those regions where this approach was adopted
  early on, it has evolved significantly over time, shifting the emphasis from
  units and centres in isolation to the roles of the networks in creating real
  integration of care. Terminology and administrative arrangements have
  varied around the country.*

- There has been increasing realisation among both commissioning and trust management that the population defined by a cancer centre, its component units and the underlying primary care and community services was the only meaningful entity within which to implement comprehensive cancer service delivery.

  *This new 'cancer geography' was not consistent with accepted organisa-
  tional boundaries in the NHS. Neither was it constant in any one area,
  reflecting different arrangements for certain services – for example, the
  location of thoracic and neurosurgery affected tertiary cancer services for
  some tumours.*

Peer reviews were initially entirely optional, but eventually became a requirement (paragraph 6.15 of the NHS Cancer Plan) in all English regions, the first
round to be completed by October 2001. They offer many potential benefits for
commissioners, clinicians and providers, through the following:

- putting the spotlight on what has been achieved, and more particularly on what has not yet been achieved
- involving the whole organisation and drawing corporate management atten-tion to cancer services in both provider and commissioning organisations
- challenging clinicians by assessing the way in which they deliver their services
- sharing experience – visitors as well as those visited learn a great deal from taking part.

The national cancer standards were developed for England partly to support the new requirement to establish processes of peer review in every region. Although these processes were not described as formal accreditation, they drew heavily on experience in the Trent Region, which does use the concepts and terminology of accreditation for its activities. Other regions, notably West Midlands, Northern and Yorkshire, and North West, also have extensive experience of running their own forms of external visitation of their cancer services, but these are not described as accreditation systems.

The approach taken by the Trent Region[24] is thus important for five main reasons.

- It was adopted by the Department of Health as representing good practice – the unofficial prototype. It was therefore influential in shaping national requirements.
- The Trent accreditation process is based on carefully drafted standards, each of which is precise and measurable, and specifies the necessary proof of compliance with those standards which must be offered during peer-review visits.
- The drafting of standards required ambiguities and imprecision of all kinds to be resolved during the formulation of standards, rather than becoming issues for variable interpretation by visitors.
- The Trent standards are based on cancer networks and define exactly how responsibilities for the various attributes of networks should be allocated for accreditation purposes.
- The roles of commissioners within the networks are included, as well as those with respect to cancer commissioning itself.

Underpinning the Trent standards is a well-worked-out concept of the organisational roles exercised by networks. The model elaborates the policy requirements of the Calman–Hine Report and the NHS Cancer Plan. It is described in some detail since it is broadly applicable. Terminology and fine detail could be altered without invalidating the fundamental concept. It set out the suggested relationships between networks and commissioners, together with the necessary ground rules. These preserve the spirit of the Calman–Hine reforms, allowing network control over service provision while at the same time having enough flexibility to make it practical for most or all configurations. They could be embodied in the national appraisal standards themselves or adopted in regional arrangements for the first or second rounds of appraisal visits. In outline, centres would be appraised as entities but would be accountable for appraisal purposes for a set of networking arrangements governing the traffic of patients to and from the centre and units. Units would be appraised as entities whose services would be under network control, but a unit could make use of more than one network.

Some of the details are given below.

The cancer centre

A cancer centre should be named, and should name the hospitals/institutions/ services that belong to it. They should belong to one centre only (and should subject themselves to the appraisal standards for one centre). They may receive referrals from other centres under certain circumstances. A centre should have one or more multidisciplinary teams (MDTs) and a disease site group (DSG) for each cancer type on the agreed service list in the standards, or should comply with the standards governing referral of that cancer type to another centre ('scope of centres' standard). Each MDT should be represented on the centre's DSG for that cancer type.

The cancer unit

A cancer unit should be named and the hospitals/institutions/services which it consists of should also be named. They should be part of only one unit and be subject to one cancer unit's appraisal. They may receive referrals from other cancer units in some circumstances. A cancer unit should have one or more MDTs for each cancer type on the list in the standards, or should comply with the standards for referral of cancer types from one unit to another unit or centre ('special case' standard). Each MDT of the unit should be represented on a disease site group for that cancer type in only one network. There may be individual agreed arrangements for referral of patients for certain tertiary services to another network. The same network need not deal with all of the MDTs for all of the different cancer sites, but if there is more than one MDT in the unit for a given single cancer type, then they should be members of the same network.

All of the chemotherapy services of a unit (solid tumour and haemato-oncology) must take part in the arrangements of the same network for the purposes of appraisal against the chemotherapy standards. A unit with radio-therapy services should agree radiotherapy referral guidelines between itself and a single named centre-based radiotherapy facility. The provision of non-surgical oncology sessions should be appraised as part of the unit's respon-sibility. It is probably impracticable to require that a unit which obtains non-surgical oncology sessions as an outreach from a centre should initially receive them all from the same centre, but this is a goal to work towards. There are already examples of units that have changed the source of their non-surgical oncologists and related services in order to fit in better with their overall network pattern and desired centre links.

The cancer network

Of all the three concepts – centre, unit and network – the network is the least structural and most functional. It is therefore rather elusive to try and define what it is, and perhaps better to define it in terms of what it should do in relation to centres and units and how it should be subjected to appraisal. However, for this approach it is essential to preserve centres and units as real entities or the whole structure becomes too loose and the ability to address successfully many of the difficult issues of Calman–Hine implementation is lost. Networks should exist to link primary and secondary services, and in this context particularly specific secondary and tertiary activities – not to provide a mechanism for inappropriate or unmanaged devolution of services.

The network functions through a series of interrelated groups which determines and controls the practice in and relationships between a centre and units. The groups are MDTs, DSGs (or network-site-specific groups; NSSGs), possibly similar groups related to other infrastructure services across the network (e.g. the delivery of chemotherapy), and a group relating to commissioners.

In order to anchor a network firmly to one named centre, the following principles should be applied.

- The lead clinician, nurse and manager for the network should be the centre leads. (Colocation with a centre has been adopted elsewhere.)
- In their referral guidelines, the DSGs for the network should recommend referral of patients to tertiary services in the named centre for that network if they are available. If they do not, the standards relating to referral to another centre apply (scope of centres).
- If practitioners have to refer to some tertiary services outside their own network, it is normally impractical for them to belong to groups relating to more than one network. They should belong to a single network and have agreed referral relationships with another if necessary for the particular service in question.

Other configurations

The Trent standards allow for centres with no related units and also for the situation where the only MDT (for a rare cancer across the whole network) exists in the centre. These variants are compatible with the above ground rules, and the necessary allowances relate mainly to fulfilling certain 'networking' functions (e.g. research, audit and relating to commissioners) where no groups spanning both centre and units exist.

Groups of services/institutions/hospitals within those named as a centre do not qualify for separate appraisal as a cancer unit. They are part of the centre, although certain services may be entirely concerned with delivering secondary (unit-type) functions to their catchment population. Groups of services/institutions/hospitals within those named as a cancer unit do not qualify for separate appraisal for centre status. If this is sought, they should seek agreement to be named as part of an established named centre and be subject to the appraisal standards for that centre/network as a whole.

These functions and the groups involved are illustrated schematically in Figures 7.1–7.3, and the principal functions are summarised. The MDTs shown in Figure 7.1 are central to all of the networks and to their operation. Linking of the different MDTs for each type of cancer is essential. With regard to the Trent standards this is achieved through a network site-specific group for a given tumour site (*see* Figure 7.2). Again, the personnel involved are schematically illustrated and the functions within the network are defined. The final

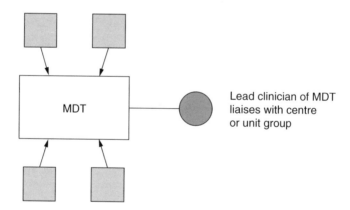

☐ Multidisciplinary practitioners for a
given tumour type within a centre or unit

MDT

Lead clinician of MDT
liaises with centre
or unit group

Functions

- The basic component of the network.
- Ensures that there is a multidisciplinary decision as to which modalities of treatment each and every patient is referred for.
- Ensures that management protocols and policies are in place and agreed by all disciplines.

Figure 7.1:   The multidisciplinary team (MDT).

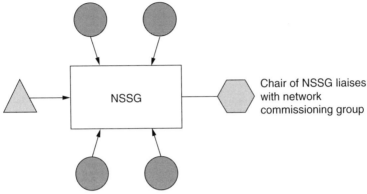

MDT leads for the given tumour type across the network
Commissioner representative

NSSG

Chair of NSSG liaises with network commissioning group

Functions

- Ensures that clinical guidelines (i.e. how a patient is managed) and referral guidelines (i.e. at which level – primary, secondary or tertiary – that patient is managed) for their particular tumour site are agreed for the network.
- Agrees a clinical minimum data set for their tumour site for the network.
- Agrees an 'approved list' of clinical trials for the network, necessary for meeting targets for clinical trial entry.

Figure 7.2: The network site-specific group (NSSG) for a given tumour site (DSG).

element is the network commissioning group (*see* Figure 7.3). All three of these examples demonstrate how detailed standards ensure that organisational issues such as networks can be drawn into accreditation, alongside service provision and clinical issues. All standards are equally capable of appraisal by peer review.

Although it is possible to use different terms to describe these bodies, and within limits to adapt the representation to suit specific circumstances, the functions described are essential for the effective network-wide management of services for particular cancers, and for the effective network commissioning of these services. The semantics of the appraisal process are probably not crucial either. Accreditation, appraisal and assessment are different terms for processes that have much in common. The key to making a success of any approach lies in the rigour with which standards are developed, clarity about the evidence necessary to assess compliance with the standards, and sound organisation of the assessment processes.

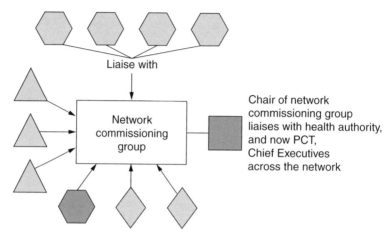

Health authority representative
Cancer unit lead clinician
Cancer centre lead clinician
NSSG chairs

Liaise with

Network commissioning group

Chair of network commissioning group liaises with health authority, and now PCT, Chief Executives across the network

Functions

• Co-ordinates commissioning for the network.
• Agrees a programme of audit projects for giving tumour sites across the network.
• Provides commissioners' input to clinical and referral guidelines.

Figure 7.3:   Network commissioning group.

The nature and role of national cancer guidance

The draft Calman–Hine Report went out for consultation in 1994, and the definitive document was published early in 1995. Both Chief Medical Officers of England and Wales at that time were clear that further advice was necessary in order to define in more detail how services for particular cancers should be delivered. A high priority was given to initiating arrangements for producing this advice in an authoritative form. Perhaps surprisingly, the Department of Health had no past experience of initiating the production of detailed evidence-based service guidance. As visualised, the guidance went beyond the conventional format of policy documents or working party reports. What was envisaged lay somewhere between broad statements of policy and the fine detail necessary for clinical guidelines. Indeed, at the same time the Department of Health was actively encouraging national professional bodies to write national clinical guidelines such as those that were produced for breast cancer (British Association of Surgical Oncology[25]) and bowel cancer (Royal College of Surgeons and Association of Coloproctologists[26]) and the equivalent SIGN (Scottish Intercollegiate Guidelines Network) guidelines in Scotland.[27]

The Department's terms of reference for the cancer guidance were couched in a general manner. They laid down three potentially conflicting parameters, namely to utilise evidence rigorously, to keep the main professions 'on board', and to take into account resource requirements. The latter was an ever present preoccupation at the time when this process was initiated. The Department of Health's first move was to establish a committee (now called the National Cancer Guidance Group) under the Chairmanship of Professor Bob Haward at Leeds University. Their expectation was that this committee would itself somehow produce the guidance. In the event, the approach taken was radically different and led to the work becoming a commissioned project working to a well-defined methodology. The committee's role is now limited to overseeing and supporting the project teams. This approach was further formalised in 2000 by the transfer of responsibility for a further series of guidance documents from the Department of Health itself to the National Institute for Clinical Excellence (NICE). They now contract for this work along precisely those lines that had previously evolved.

The initial task was to agree how this work should be done, and to select, adapt or devise an appropriate methodology. Woolf[28] described four broad types of methodology as suitable for clinical guideline production. These were as follows:

- informal consensus development
- formal consensus development
- evidence-based guideline development
- explicit guideline development.

Informal consensus development is the process by which an expert group, often dominated by a particular discipline with interests in the area concerned, produces recommendations. This is achieved without either a systematic process for searching, reviewing and presenting evidence, or any prior rules or processes for the guideline development itself.

Formal consensus development encompasses a variety of methods that all have common formalised processes for obtaining and testing the views of invited experts, who are key to the process. However, whilst expert opinion is utilised in a carefully structured manner, the research evidence itself is neither searched nor assembled according to rigorous techniques such as those now used by the Cochrane Collaboration.

Evidence-based guideline development is the antithesis of the formal consensus approach in that the emphasis is on proper methods for searching, extracting, reviewing and presenting published research evidence. There is no clear-cut process for the translation of this material into guidelines.

The final method, and the one selected, is *explicit guideline development*, in which both the approach to evidence and the use of an explicit process are encompassed in one approach. The advantage of an explicit process, described by Grimshawe,[29,30] is that it is most likely to lead to valid recommendations, since it is not dominated by the interests of any one professional group and it draws on both expert opinion and systematic reviews of the research evidence.

Because there was no practical existing model that suited the needs of the project, a methodology was developed specifically to produce this guidance. This work was carried out by members of the national committee, with input from the Centre for Reviews and Dissemination at York University and external expert advice from Professor David Eddy,[31] who is experienced in clinical guideline development for the American College of Physicians. The resulting methodology was finalised during the production of the first guidance document, for breast cancer, which was published in 1996. The method has remained essentially unchanged, although some refinements were added in subsequent documents.

Guidance was also published for colorectal cancer in 1997, lung cancer in 1998, gynaecological cancers in 1999 and upper gastrointestinal cancers in 2000. Further new guidance was commissioned by NICE (in 2000) to be published in 2002–03 to cover urological cancers, haemato-oncology and head and neck cancers. In addition, and using the same methodology, there is to be generic guidance on supportive care (across all sites of cancer), to be published in 2002/03. The updating of the early cancer guidance reports is now scheduled, with the first update of the breast cancer guidance due in 2002. It is now anticipated that following publication of each update there will be a new version of that guidance specifically written to meet the needs of users. This reflects the increasing recognition of the importance of informing those who may need services in a transparent and straightforward manner.

Each set of guidance is published in three separate parts. The recommendations are set out in the *Manual*. This is backed up by a more substantial document summarising the *Research Evidence*. The whole is summarised in a shortened version called the *GP Summary*. In addition, York University publishes a separate summary of the research evidence in their series of *Effective Health Care Bulletins*.

Evidence reviews are vital not only to underpin the recommendations but also to inform users. Those using the guidance must be able to see for themselves how comprehensive or limited the evidence was for any one topic area, and hence how solid the recommendations were. This transparency is essential for guideline users, otherwise the applicability of the recommendations cannot be evaluated in any way.

The process of formulating recommendations inevitably involves judgements. These have to take into account all forms of evidence, such as expert opinion, published research evidence, data from audits and descriptive studies of services. Judgements inevitably also reflect the importance to the NHS of recommendations on any particular point. Reconciling evidence of all types and from varied sources is far from simple. In large measure this is because the nature and strength of such evidence vary, and there are often gaps in crucial areas. Some recommendations do rest solidly on accumulated evidence from large-scale randomised trials and authoritative overviews such as those for breast cancer.[32] Recommendations in these areas are therefore relatively straightforward and uncontroversial. However, the issues on which commissioners, providers of care and lead clinicians for particular services need advice are often in the area of service configuration and organisation. Which personnel should be involved? What work should be done at which point in the system? How does the whole fit best together, taking into account wider service implications? Without a service model for each site-specific cancer or service group of cancers, the guidance is unlikely to succeed as a useful initiative.

The evidence base for recommendations in these areas tends to come from prospective and retrospective observational studies, from major audits, from cancer registries, and in North America from administrative databases. This type of evidence is difficult to put together because of differences in study design and the inevitable pragmatic way in which the studies were conducted (e.g. they may have drawn on data that were available rather than ideal). Such evidence can be searched, assembled and categorised as well as any other.

The Centre for Reviews and Dissemination at York University manages the process of assembling evidence for the national cancer guidance. This organisation was created to undertake the systematic assembly of evidence and its dissemination to support NHS decision making. Some of the reviews are contracted out to appropriate expert groups, normally the Cochrane Group for that particular cancer, if one exists. The management of evidence reviews is a complex and iterative process. Fresh evidence problems are identified throughout the editorial process for each guidance document. Only when the guidance manual is finished can the evidence review itself be finalised and assembled in a publishable form. Evidence reviews are not therefore static summaries, but require questions to be posed and hypotheses put forward which can then be tested independently by the evidence reviewers.

The guidance project captures expert opinion early in the methodology through the first two stages of a four-stage development process (*see* Figure 7.4). This commences with a residential event, known as a *proposal generating event*, with a mix of clinical disciplines and some patients. This produces a series of proposals which are expressed in a specific format. These are then tested on a wider multidisciplinary audience through a mechanism akin to peer review.

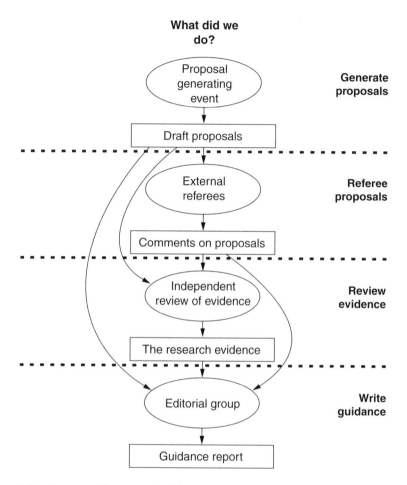

Figure 7.4: Cancer guidance methodology.

Thus it is possible for evidence reviewers to identify the issues which expert opinion believes to be important. The peer review often demonstrates which proposals are broadly accepted or controversial. There may be alternative or competing ideas within any one set of proposals, which itself demonstrates a lack of consensus among those concerned.

The topics covered in each cancer guidance report vary slightly with the actual service issues relevant to the specific forms of cancer that are covered in each document. The issues generally involve key recommendations for commissioners, with sections on access to care, diagnosis, staging, initial treatment, and the management of recurrent disease and palliative care. Within each topic the format is consistent. Recommendations are set out first, followed by the anticipated benefits, a brief rehearsal of the nature of the evidence, a section describing measurement (i.e. suggested measures which might indicate whether or not the recommendations were being implemented) and finally a section on resource implications. All of the documents are prefaced by an introduction which sets out the healthcare epidemiology of the disease. Detailed lists of everyone who has been involved are included. Transparency with regard to the latter issue is important if there is to be confidence in the outcome. It should be quite clear to users who has (and who has not) taken part in any way. It is normal practice to list all those who were sent copies of the proposals for peer review, not simply those who responded. Typically the response rate to peer review is about 40%.

The two most recent guidance documents (those for gynaecological cancers and upper gastrointestinal cancers) included economic reviews[33] (commissioned from the School of Health and Related Research at Sheffield University) setting out the resource consequences of implementing the main recommendations. There are substantial resource implications arising from the service reconfigurations recommended in the guidance for intermediate-frequency cancers. Reconfiguring of services inevitably leads to developments in some locations and a consequent decline in activities in others. In addition, some resource implications reflect under-utilisation of diagnostic or treatment modalities, despite clear evidence of benefit. Where the role of particular diagnostic or treatment modalities has been recommended for expansion, the implications of adopting them are also costed. These economic studies show that costs vary considerably from one setting to another.

One feature of the recommendations in more recent guidance documents has been the extent to which those recommendations identify issues for local resolution within the cancer networks. This reflects the growing emphasis on the role of these networks. Although it is not defensible to subvert major recommendations in the guidance, there are many issues for which there is no simple right answer for the management of individual patients. Recommendations have to be applied in ways that make operational sense. These issues are exemplified by the key recommendations in the upper gastrointestinal guidance (*see* Figure 7.4 and Box 7.3), where five out of the six key recommendations require agreements to be reached within cancer networks if the revised service model is to be implemented effectively.

Box 7.3:   Upper gastrointestinal cancer guidance: key recommendations

- All hospitals which intend to provide services for patients with upper gastrointestinal cancer should be fully involved in appropriate cancer networks which include interlinked cancer centres and cancer units. Each region should review proposals for these services, to ensure that the proposed local arrangements reflect the recommendations in this guidance manual accurately.

- There should be documented local referral policies for diagnostic services for suspected upper gastrointestinal cancer. These should be jointly agreed between general practitioners in primary care groups and trusts, and appropriate specialists in local hospitals and cancer units and centres in each network.
- Specialist treatment teams should be established at appropriate cancer centres or units. Oesophago-gastric cancer teams should aim to draw patients from populations of more than one million; pancreatic cancer teams should aim to draw patients from populations of two to four million.
- There should be clear documented policies for referral of patients between hospitals, and for processes by which clinicians in local hospitals seek advice from specialist treatment teams about the management of individual patients for whom referral may not be appropriate.
- Palliative support and specialist care should be available to all who need it. This will require effective co-ordination and communication between primary care, social and voluntary services, local palliative care teams, hospital services and those who provide specialist advice and interventions.
- Monitoring systems using common data sets should be established throughout each cancer network to audit patient management, key communications, referral processes and key outcomes of treatment.

Because the guidance defines the MDTs necessary at the different levels in the service for the management of particular cancers, the guidance recommendations are particularly amenable to incorporation into standards for peer review. A programme of rolling out the guidance recommendations for MDT configuration and functioning for each cancer type as additions to the *Manual of Cancer Services Standards* is planned in parallel to the National Cancer Guidance Programme. The guidance lists a series of measures that are important to the assessment of services, or the monitoring of implementation of particular aspects of the guidance. This can be easily utilised, feeding into the shaping of audit agendas, particularly collaborative audits within networks, and contributing to national debate about the data that should be enshrined in data sets for each site of cancer. The explicit recommendations about the professions and disciplines required for service delivery within each network facilitate manpower planning and training.

The guidance is complementary to Department of Health policies and targets dealing with access to cancer care. The two-week wait initiative and similar new standards set out in the NHS Cancer Plan for the interval between urgent referral and the start of treatment draw on the guidance. This specifies who should be managing these diseases at the various service levels. It also specifies how diagnosis, assessment, staging and decision making about treatment should be undertaken. Thus pathways of care are broadly defined by cancer guidance.

Although the guidance was originally intended for commissioners, this was in part because of the NHS culture that prevailed at the time when it was initiated. Market thinking was still current, and the orthodoxy was that guidance directed towards providers was not the right way to shape services. The modern application of the guidance is likely to be increasingly through decisions taken within cancer networks, of which commissioning is only one element. Within commissioning it is unclear how the responsibilities of primary care trusts will develop to absorb those of former health authorities. In any case, cancer networks will continue to require a co-ordinated and strategic approach from their commissioners, whoever they are and however many. The new cancer geography has established itself as a structural fact of life, which is likely to be very stable. As a result, organisational manipulation, re-organisations or mergers do not readily affect it.

The title of the guidance, *Improving Outcomes in . . .* , reflects a fundamental concern to promote those changes, with the realistic expectation that services organised in the ways that are recommended are more likely to produce good outcomes than the service patterns that pre-date the guidance. Although outcomes in cancer are often dominated by survival, these documents are concerned with wider outcomes. These include patient satisfaction with services, and qualitative issues for patients, such as morbidity resulting from different aspects of care and quality of life. Past research has shown huge variability in the processes of care within the UK (as in other countries), and between the UK and other countries in Europe and North America.

Is there evidence that this cancer guidance has met the expectations of those for whom it has been produced? Sadly, there has been no independent evaluation of the national cancer guidance, despite the fact that the National Cancer Guidance Group has urged the commissioning of such an evaluation. The Centre for Health Economics in York undertook a limited commissioner focus group evaluation of the guidance (copies of which are available on request), although this has not yet been published. This evaluation was extremely positive among the commissioners for whom the guidance was intended. The level of anticipation of each new document, and the surge of activity across the NHS that follows publication, suggests that the guidance provides something of real value.

The combination of the Calman–Hine Report and the site-specific guidance has clearly generated changes in the provision of services. Long-term improvements in survival, if they have occurred, will take some years to be manifested in national statistics. There is some indirect evidence from surveys of processes of care. For example, following the Calman–Hine Report in 1995, and

Table 7.1: Year of formation of breast teams in England*

Year started	Number of teams	
1980–84	2	0.2 per annum
1985–89	6	1.2 per annum
1990–94	19	3.8 per annum
1995	9	
1996	12	
1997	15	
1998	10	
1999	8	

*Data from study not yet published: Haward R, West M, Borril C, Amir Z and Sainsbury R (2002) Stratified random sample (by NHS region and caseload) of breast teams.

the national cancer guidance for breast cancer in 1996, there was a surge in the formation of new breast MDTs. Table 7.1 shows the year in which regular team meetings began for a random sample of breast teams in England stratified by NHS region. There was also a significant rise[21] in the number of non-surgical oncologists working in cancer units, as required in the Calman–Hine Report.

The gathering momentum in the early 1990s in response to the belief that 'something had to be done' to address serious shortcomings in UK cancer care led to the Calman–Hine Report. This has proved to be the catalyst for a hugely influential process of change. It has caused real changes in the organisation and clinical delivery of cancer services, sustained and reinforced by the publication five years later of the NHS Cancer Plan, with genuine additional resources. Despite these documents, the crucial problem of how best to configure services to achieve the best outcomes for patients with each site of cancer, or service group of cancers, still had to be confronted. The UK had evolved a very fragmented approach to many potentially curative or complex interventions, characterised by inadequate specialisation, low volumes at clinician and hospital level, and a failure to make management decisions in a fully multidisciplinary way in many cases.

In breast,[34] colorectum[35] and lung cancer,[36] this has largely been addressed by the guidance recommendations directed towards cancer-unit-based MDTs. For intermediate-frequency cancers, such as gynaecological[37] and upper gastrointestinal cancers,[38] more service centralisation is recommended. Without clear site-specific guidance the forces opposing or passively resisting change in this state of affairs may well have succeeded in retaining the historically unsatisfactory pattern of service delivery. The cancer guidance has been the necessary mechanism for this to be challenged constructively. The guidance has set out a modern service model in each case, which is supported by careful reviews of the relevant evidence. This has enabled commissioners and now cancer networks to address *how to bring about necessary change*, and not to become bogged down in debating *what if any changes need to be made*, in their areas.

References

1   Department of Health (1999) *Working for Patients*. The Stationery Office, London.

2   Sheaff WR and Peel VJ (1993) *Best Practice in Health Care Commissioning*. Churchill Livingstone, London.

3   Department of Health (1993) *Managing the New NHS: a background document*. Department of Health, London.

4   NHS Executive (1998) *National Specialist Commissioning Advisory Group: applications for designation and central funding of highly specialised services*. HSC 1998/098. Department of Health, London.

5   NHS Executive (1998) *Commissioning in the New NHS*. HSC 1998/198. Department of Health, London.

6   Glennester H, Matsaganis M and Owens P (1992) *A Foothold for Fundholding*. King's Fund Institute, London.

7   British Medical Association (1993) *Fundholding: an introductory guide*. British Medical Association, London.

8   Department of Health (1999) *Primary Care Groups: taking the next steps*. HSC 1999/246, LAC (99)40. Department of Health, London; also available on http://www.doh.gov.uk/coinh.htm

9   Dixon M (2000/01) NHS organisations: primary care groups and trusts. In: P Merry (ed.) *Wellard NHS Handbook 2000/01* (15e). JMH Publishing, London.

10 Department of Health (1995) *Policy Framework for Commissioning Cancer Services: a Report by the Expert Advisory Group on Cancer to the Chief Medical Officers of England and Wales*. HMSO, London.

11 NHS Cervical Screening Programme (1996) *Quality Assurance Guidelines for the Cervical Screening Programme: report of a working party*. NHS Executive, London.

12 Department of Health (1984) *Acute Hospital Services for Cancer Patients, HN (84)23, and the Report of the Working Group: the Bagshawe Report*. HMSO, London.

13 Department of Health (2000) *The NHS Cancer Plan*. Department of Health, London.

14 Sant M, Capocaccia R, Verdecchia A *et al.* (1995) Comparisons of colon-cancer survival among European countries: the Eurocare Study. *Int J Cancer*. 63: 43–8.

15 Sainsbury R, Rider L, Smith A, Macadam A and the Yorkshire Breast Cancer Group (1995) Does it matter where you live? Treatment variation for breast cancer in Yorkshire. *Br J Cancer*. 71: 1275–8.

16 Bull AD, Biffin AHB, Mella J et al. (1997) Colorectal cancer pathology reporting: a regional audit. *J Clin Pathol.* **50**: 138–42.

17 Gillis CR and Hole DJ (1996) Survival outcome of care by specialist surgeons in breast cancer: a study of 3786 patients in the west of Scotland. *BMJ.* **312**: 145–8.

18 Selby P, Gillis C and Haward R (1996) Benefits from specialised cancer care. *Lancet.* **348**: 313–18.

19 Junor EJ, Hole DJ and Gillis CR (1994) Management of ovarian cancer: referral to a multidisciplinary team matters. *Br J Cancer.* **70**: 363–70.

20 Haward RA (1995) Establishing cancer units. *Br J Cancer.* **72**: 531–4.

21 Scott E, Haward R and Wilkinson J (1998) Professional approaches. *Health Serv J.* **23 April**: 30–31.

22 Haward R and Amir Z (2000) Progress in establishing non-surgical oncology within English cancer units. *Br J Cancer.* **83**: 284–6.

23 NHS Executive (2000) *Manual of Cancer Service Standards.* Department of Health, London.

24 NHS Executive (2000) *Professional Standards for Accreditation of Cancer Centres and Cancer Units (Second Round).* NHS Executive, Trent.

25 British Association of Surgical Oncology (BASO) (1995) Guidelines for surgeons in the management of symptomatic breast disease in the United Kingdom. *Eur J Surg Oncol.* **21 (Supplement A)**: 1–13.

26 Royal College of Surgeons of England and the Association of Coloproctology of Great Britain and Ireland (1996) *Guidelines for the Management of Colorectal Cancer.* Royal College of Surgeons of England and the Association of Coloproctology of Great Britain and Ireland, London.

27 Scottish Cancer Therapy Network (1997) *Colorectal Cancer: a national clinical guideline recommended for use in Scotland.* Publication No 16. Scottish Cancer Therapy Network, Edinburgh.

28 Woolf S (1992) Practice guidelines: a new reality in medicine. *Arch Intern Med.* **152**: 946–52.

29 Grimshaw JM and Russell IT (1993) Effect of clinical guidelines on medical practice: a systematic review of rigorous evaluations. *Lancet.* **342**: 1317–22.

30 Grimshaw J, Eccles M and Russell I (1995) Developing clinically valid practice guidelines. *J Eval Clin Pract.* **1**: 37–48.

31 Eddy DM (1992) *Assessing Health Practices and Designing Practice Policies.* American College of Physicians, Philadelphia, PA.

32 Early Breast Cancer Trialists' Collaborative Group (1992) Systemic treatment of early breast cancer by hormonal, cytotoxic or immune therapy. *Lancet.* **339**: 1–15, 71–85.

33 Ward S, Clayton E, Brennan A and Warren E (2000) *Analysis of the Potential Impact of Guidance on the Management of Upper Gastrointestinal Cancers.* School of Health and Related Research, University of Sheffield, Sheffield.

34 Cancer Guidance Subgroup of the Clinical Outcomes Group (1996) *Improving Outcomes in Breast Cancer.* Department of Health, London (Manual Cat. Nos 96CC0021 and Research Evidence 96CC0022).

35 Cancer Guidance Subgroup of the Clinical Outcomes Group (1997). *Improving Outcomes in Colorectal Cancer.* Department of Health, London (Manual 97CV0119 and Research Evidence 97CC0120).

36 Cancer Guidance Subgroup of the Clinical Outcomes Group (1998) *Improving Outcomes in Lung Cancer.* Department of Health, London (Manual 97CC122 and Research Evidence 97CC123).

37 National Cancer Guidance Group (1999) *Improving Outcomes in Gynaecological Cancers.* Department of Health, London (Manual 16149 and Research Evidence 16150).

38 National Cancer Guidance Group (2000) *Improving Outcomes in Upper Gastrointestinal Cancers.* Department of Health, London (Manual 23180 and Research Evidence 23943).

Note: many current Department of Health cancer documents are available on its website at http://www.doh.gov.uk/cancer/

CHAPTER 8

Cancer in primary care

Nicholas Summerton

Introduction

The recently published NHS Cancer Plan sets very high standards for cancer services throughout England.[1] This is to be applauded, and for those of us with an interest in primary care oncology it is encouraging that the central role of primary care is being re-emphasised. The NHS Cancer Plan proposes that each primary care trust should have a lead cancer clinician, and it seems likely that such individuals will also have the opportunity to become more closely involved in the further development of cancer networks.

Primary care has not traditionally been seen as essential to the planning and provision of cancer services. However, building on the suggestions that were first made in the Calman–Hine Report,[2] there now seems to be a genuine acknowledgement that the primary care perspective cannot be ignored. The general practitioner (GP) and the primary care team have important and growing roles in all aspects of the cancer journey from primary prevention through screening to diagnosis, treatment and continuing care. Matching the broader perspective of the NHS Cancer Plan, the GP is also increasingly concerned with public health priorities such as healthcare commissioning and health inequalities.

There is much evidence that general practitioners could serve individual cancer patients better. According to Nylenna, one-third of patients are often not even recognised as having a malignancy by their general practitioner,[3] and in a recent survey in Lothian, only one-fifth of practices maintained a cancer register[4]. A study of cancer patients in Canada revealed that although well over half thought that their family doctor had been involved in diagnosis, only 26% considered that their GP had any role in their treatment[5]. Furthermore, less than 60% thought that their family doctor was aware of their current problems, and less than one-third had an appointment to see their doctor in the near future. It is often very difficult for the general practitioner to become involved with a patient's care again after a long period of separation. Cancer patient attendance at Accident and Emergency departments has also been repeatedly cited as a marker of inadequacies in cancer recognition and management in primary care. According to Hargarten and colleagues, 5.3% of new cancer patients may present in this way, and such individuals are invariably older, with more frequent metastatic disease and a poor prognosis.[6]

Diagnosis and referral

Delayed cancer diagnosis can have adverse effects on patient survival.[7] It may also increase patient distress and disability, as later-stage cancers often require more extensive and aggressive treatment. For many patients, the general practitioner's most fundamental role is being able to act appropriately when they attend with a symptom about which they are concerned. In a recent review of complaints about general practitioners received by the Medical Defence Union, failure of or delay in diagnosis accounted for 28% of the notifications.[8] The most frequent clinical condition associated with such diagnostic failure or delay was missed malignancy. On the other hand, over-diagnosis or unnecessarily excessive testing (diagnostic inefficiency) can lead to both physical and psychological damage. Furthermore, at a public health level, all types of diagnostic errors have cost implications. Introducing better evidence into the assessment of patients within general practice could lead to better targeting of resources and, for individual patients, a more rational and appropriate balance between benefits and harm.

The Eurocare programme has highlighted the potential for improvements in cancer recognition as assessed by the stage at patient presentation for definitive treatment.[9] The pathway to care in patients with, for example, colorectal cancer is often very complex. In the absence of a screening programme it involves a combination of patient and professional reactions to symptoms of possible oncological significance. However, compared with the UK, it seems that our colleagues in The Netherlands are receiving patients at an earlier Duke's stage, with consequent improvements in survival. Other evidence from a cross-sectional study in certain North American states suggests that primary care provision is important with regard to earlier cancer diagnosis. Roetzheim and colleagues have demonstrated that the supply of primary care physicians is significantly correlated with the stage at diagnosis of patients with colorectal cancer. As the supply of primary care physicians increased, the odds of late-stage diagnosis decreased.[10]

With regard to earlier cancer recognition, the general practitioner has a particularly onerous task. Many patients often choose to avoid consulting their GP about potentially significant symptoms of cancer, as a result of ignorance, anxiety, embarrassment or denial. Others may make an initial approach to a nurse, pharmacist or even the doctor's receptionist. Once they have finally reached the general practitioner, the doctor is faced with a very difficult sifting role.

Many patients with cancer present with common symptoms such as persistent cough or non-specific abdominal pain, yet very few patients whom GPs see with such problems turn out to have malignant disease. The typical UK general practitioner will only encounter, on average, eight to nine new cases of cancer each year.[11]

In May 1999, the UK Government announced that all cases of suspected cancer would be seen by a cancer specialist within two weeks.[12] Many such specialists expressed immediate concern that such a policy could actually have adverse effects by potentially prolonging waiting times for patients referred non-urgently and for those with problems other than cancer. Therefore, as part of the process of managing the two-week wait initiative, the Department of Health asked Professor Richards, Sainsbury Professor of Palliative Medicine at St Thomas's Hospital, London, to lead a programme in order to develop referral guidelines for general practitioners. The stated aim of the guidance was to 'facilitate appropriate referral between primary and secondary care for patients whom a GP suspects may have cancer and who therefore require urgent assessment by a specialist'. Equally, it was hoped that the guidelines would help GPs to identify those patients who are unlikely to have cancer and who may be appropriately observed in a primary care setting or may require non-urgent referral to hospital.

In generating any guideline, it is necessary to be systematic in the way in which the evidence is collected and aggregated, as well as the way in which values are incorporated into the recommendations. None of us who have been involved in the cancer referral guidelines initiative would claim that the work matched up to the highest standards of evidence-based guideline development.[13] The time available simply did not allow an explicit and systematic review of the available literature to be undertaken. Moreover, a subsequent systematic review by the author (funded by the Royal College of General Practitioners Scientific Foundation Board) has revealed very little high-quality or applicable evidence in the majority of areas of cancer recognition in primary care. Other reviewers have identified specific deficiencies in, for example, the relationship between chronic cough and lung cancer[14] and that between haematuria and urological malignancies.[15,16]

In terms of incorporating primary care values into the referral guidelines, Professor Richards actively sought the involvement of a number of general practitioners in the guideline groups. In addition, written responses were invited (and received) from a number of general practitioners, and a series of roadshows was conducted around the country. Although this activity served to enhance the primary care perspective, the approach was far from systematic. It is interesting to note that key omissions from the guidelines point to an inability to appreciate that patients present to general practitioners with symptoms, and that these early symptoms may not easily fit into a site-specific cancer grouping. Significant evidence from The Netherlands in relation to the non-specific diagnosis of 'intra-abdominal malignancy' was brought to the attention of tumour groups, but was not considered.[17] Furthermore, one of the most popular chapters among general practitioners in the book *Diagnosing Cancer in Primary Care* has been the final chapter on 'non-specific features of malignant disease' – perhaps because this takes a more generalist and symptom-oriented approach.[11]

I believe that the Department of Health is quite correct in highlighting the GP responsibility for cancer recognition, but their solution requires considerable further development. In the longer term it is clear that consensus guidelines written predominantly by consultants and based on inadequate or inapplicable evidence are simply not the best way to guide GPs in the rational assessment of the types of patients whom they encounter and in the settings where they work. Clearly there is now an urgent need for primary care to seize the initiative and to build on the referral guidelines project and use it as an opportunity to address the inadequacies in the available evidence. Some initial steps were taken in the early 1960s, when Ian McWhinney published practice-based clinical research examining the early diagnosis of cancer,[18] and this was followed four years later by Starey's work on the diagnosis and treatment of cancer in his practice.[19] However, in the last 20 to 30 years, it seems that primary care research has moved away from a clinical orientation. In 1995, Owen lamented the fact that medical research has yet to address in any meaningful manner what symptoms and signs indicated in primary care are useful in predicting a certain disease, which are not useful, and which will rule out a disease.[20]

Primary care researchers must be encouraged to generate information in order to improve the timeliness, accuracy and efficiency of cancer recognition by primary care staff. In view of the problems with selection bias first encountered by McWhinney,[18] and subsequently examined by others,[21] it has become clear that a community-based approach is the most sensible way to address such questions, but it will require significant funding, organisation and collaboration. It is reassuring that the need for such large-scale and fundamental clinical research has now been highlighted by the House of Commons Select Committee on Science and Technology.[22] Furthermore, the establishment of a National Cancer Research Network as part of the NHS Cancer Plan presents a golden opportunity to develop this type of large-scale clinical epidemiology. However, in supporting such a development there are a number of key considerations that must be appreciated.

The patient spectrum

As a result of the different prevalences of cancers between primary care and secondary care, the probability of cancer should a 'test' (i.e. a symptom, sign or investigation) be positive (the positive predictive value) would not be the same in primary care. Unfortunately, misunderstandings about the impact of disease prevalence in a population on the predictive value of a test have led to fundamental disagreements between general practitioners and specialists with regard to the usefulness of all types of clinical discriminant information (i.e. symptoms, signs and investigations).[21,23] This is particularly the case for cancer, where the majority of textbooks and guidelines assume that such information can simply be transposed directly from secondary to primary care.

To compound matters further, patients in primary care present to their doctors with symptoms that are generally less clearly defined than those of patients attending the specialist service. By the time the patient reaches the clinic, symptoms will have evolved and the patient will also have had more time to reflect on his or her story. The underlying disease process is also evolutionary, and it is well known that the symptoms of early-stage cancers are different to those of later stages. In many ways a GP has to deal with a first draft, whereas the consultant gets the edited typescript.

The diagnostic dilemma is well illustrated by the 'symptom pyramid' (*see* Figure 8.1). In the community or in primary care, cough is much less likely to indicate an underlying lung cancer than it would be in a specialist chest clinic. In addition, as patients move up the pyramid and time passes, symptoms and pathologies develop and the picture becomes much clearer. It is also important to appreciate that selective referral practices to secondary care will be influenced not only by the patient's symptoms and signs, but also by their age, sex and comorbidities. In short, the spectrum of patients who are encountered by specialists will be quite distinct from that of patients who are seen in primary care.

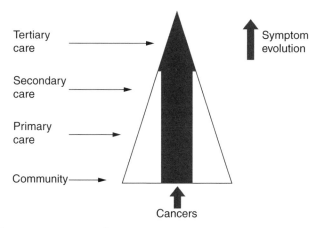

Figure 8.1:   The symptom pyramid.

The primary care perspective

General practitioners who need to make onward referrals for definitive diagnosis and treatment are often placed in the unenviable position of balancing the conflicting demands and expectations of patients, consultants, primary care trusts and professional organisations. As indicated earlier, they are always concerned not to miss a serious or important condition in a patient, but they also wish to avoid unnecessary referral.

Traditional teaching disseminated from specialist centres is focused on consultant encounters. This educational 'programming' is further underpinned by a natural tendency of consultants to judge general practitioner referral practices from their specialist perspective. Thus patients with symptoms of possible oncological significance who are encountered by a general practitioner will (over a period of time) fall into one of the following four groups:

1   those who are referred on immediately and turn out to have significant disease (the 'good GP' group)
2   those who are initially missed and who reach the specialist later than is ideal (the 'poor GP' group)
3   those who are referred but do not require specialist treatment (the 'over-cautious GP')
4   those who are not referred and who do not require specialist treatment (the 'gatekeeper role' of the GP).

Specialists who provide feedback to general practitioners as well as clinical training for medical students and general practitioner registrars obviously never encounter the vast majority of patients who are seen by general practitioners (group 4 above). Their educational activity is distorted towards addressing perceived inadequacies in groups 2 and 3. Unfortunately, there is often little appreciation that the information which is available (and reiterated in the teaching sessions) is not the most appropriate information to assist general practitioners in making an initial referral decision.

Decisions that are made in general practices are also of a different nature to those of hospital specialists. For the general practitioner, the type of decision is more dichotomous and functional (i.e. referral vs. non-referral, serious vs. less serious), rather than pathological. The general practitioner also has to cope with a greater degree of uncertainty, as the level of risk that a GP is required to accommodate is quite different to that which is acceptable to a consultant. It would be unusual for a patient to be discharged from a clinic without undergoing some form of investigation. In general practice, the vast majority of patients with, for example, episodic abdominal pain will be reassured on the basis of history and examination alone.

Revisiting the medical history

In primary care, where there is necessarily a much greater dependence on the medical history, there is a need to re-examine the history in terms of both its depth and its breadth. According to Ryle, cited by McWhinney, 'there is no symptom as yet adequately explored'[24] and, for example, there is a need to be much clearer about what is meant by the phrase 'change in bowel habit'. Furthermore, apart from the use of 'traditional items' in the clinical history, it seems that certain pieces of clinical information which are more readily and uniquely available to primary care might have significant weights of evidence that would aid the identification of malignancy in primary care settings. For example, in 1966 Pereira-Gray commented on the importance of behaviour change in indicating a likelihood of malignancy.[25] One specific example that is often cited is a recent decision to stop smoking. In a large cohort study, Nylenna noted that the patient's fear of cancer was an important predictor of malignancy.[26] In 1988, Olesen examined the pattern of attendance in patients for three years prior to the diagnosis of cervical carcinoma, and noted that significantly more patients than controls had had no doctor contact.[27] Dynamic evidence, such as the addition of new features or the persistence of or changes in the characteristics of previous problems, is particularly relevant within general practice where patients are assessed over a period of time. In addition, in a low-prevalence population, clusters of items in the medical history will most probably be of greater relevance than single items of information. Symptom enquiry may also need to be approached differently, as 'medically unsocialised' community-based patients tend to be less familiar with medical terminology than patients who are attending clinics.

The need to enhance clinical examination skills

In parallel with the generation of applicable clinical history discriminators, there is also a need to enhance clinical examination skills in collaboration with appropriate specialists. Recent work has indicated that a patient's likelihood of undergoing a rectal examination is completely unrelated to their prior probability.[28] Although the incidence of colorectal cancer rises rapidly after the age of 50 years, Summerton and Paes have demonstrated that in patients with rectal bleeding or a change in bowel habit there was no difference between rectal and abdominal examinations in individuals over the age of 50 years compared with those under the age of 50 years. Other workers have demonstrated deficiencies in clinical breast evaluation skills[29] and the ability to detect melanomas[30] among general practitioners.

Cancer care

Increasingly, GPs and other primary healthcare professionals are becoming involved in cancer treatment. Cancer therapy has traditionally been the province of site-specific specialists or oncologists. However, primary care clinicians are gradually and necessarily becoming more involved in the management of patients with curable as well as incurable disease. Many of the growing number of hormonal agents for treating breast cancer and prostate cancer are increasingly administered in primary care.[31]

In many situations, routine clinical evaluation remains important for identifying those patients who can benefit most from curative therapy. Determining whether patients with lung cancer have metastatic disease is crucial to optimum management, and invaluable information can be provided by the general practitioner. A meta-analysis by Silvestri and colleagues has revealed that clinical assessment is a very powerful tool in screening for metastatic disease (negative predictive value greater than 97%).[32] A negative clinical evaluation based on the criteria listed in Box 8.1 should reassure the clinician that the likelihood of obtaining a positive brain or abdominal CT scan or radionuclide bone scan is small.

Box 8.1: Clinical findings that suggest metastatic disease

Symptoms elicited in history
    Constitutional – weight loss greater than 10 pounds
    Musculoskeletal – focal skeletal pain
    Neurological – headaches, syncope, seizures, extremity weakness,
       recent change in mental status

Signs found on physical examination
    Lymphadenopathy (greater than 1 cm)
    Hoarseness, superior vena cava syndrome
    Bone tenderness
    Hepatomegaly (greater than 13 cm)
    Focal neurological signs, papilloedema
    Soft tissue mass

Routine laboratory tests
    Haematocrit less than 40% in males
    Haematocrit less than 35% in females
    Elevated alkaline phosphatase, gamma glutamyl transferase,
       serum glutamic oxaloacetic transaminase

GPs can also provide specialists with invaluable information to assist them in planning a patient's care, such as background information on the patient's social circumstances, support available, and their psychological state, as well as comorbidities. In a Dutch study of 34 000 newly diagnosed cancer patients, comorbid conditions were present in over half of those patients over the age of 60 years. This was especially likely among patients with lung, kidney, stomach, bladder and prostate cancer.[33] Such comorbidity often means that the patient needs tailormade medical care, with management guidelines being adapted appropriately.

General practitioners and nurse practitioners are now becoming involved in 'intermediate'-stage investigations such as endoscopy and ultrasonography. The recent rapid advances in molecular biology also open up the future possibility of general practitioners undertaking 'near-patient' testing for genetic markers for cancers in a variety of body fluids.

In the acute phase of cancer management, primary care staff can assume important roles in relation to both supportive care and shared care. The support can be broad-ranging, seeking to enhance the patient's social, physical and psychological well-being. In many situations such support may even extend to involve the whole family in terms of addressing their enhanced risk of cancer. There are a variety of models of shared care, with the precise arrangements being determined by the nature of the cancer as well as the commitment and enthusiasm of the primary healthcare team. In some cases, such as the management of basal-cell carcinoma, GPs may even be entirely responsible for the patient's management. Many patients with chronic lymphatic leukaemia die with the disease, rather than from it, and the local haematologist often needs to provide only a minimum level of input.

Even in situations where the patient's care is predominantly undertaken in specialist settings (e.g. using chemotherapy, radiotherapy or biological therapy), it is essential that GPs have some knowledge of the key side-effects and complications of the treatments that are being used. Neutropenic sepsis is a major short-term hazard and the main cause of treatment-related death associated with cancer chemotherapy. Neutropenia occurs after most such treatment, and may also be a problem if there is irradiation of large areas of the spine. It is also necessary to be aware of the longer-term consequences of cancer treatment. For example, as most patients with testicular cancer who receive chemotherapy are curable, it is essential not to forget the possible effects of platinum-based treatments on fertility or increasing the risk of leukaemia.[31]

Some aspects of cancer treatment are self-evidently beneficial, such as the prompt recognition of treatment side-effects, or ensuring that there is effective three-way communication between the patient, the general practitioner and the specialist.[34] However, in developing a primary care role in cancer treatment, it is important to consider the capacity of primary care and to guard against any downgrading of the generalist role. Too much GP specialisation may lead to opportunity costs, with the loss of some important aspects of standard care. It is already accepted that patients with chronic disease are often not managed as well as other patients in terms of preventative activities, as the focus is primarily on their chronic illness.[35] There is good evidence that encouraging smoking cessation can, on its own, have important positive effects on a cancer patient's outcome, and this is well provided in a traditional primary care setting.[36] General practitioners and primary healthcare teams who neglect the old in favour of the new and novel may not necessarily produce the improved patient outcomes that they desire.

Suggested service reconfigurations, with a shift of secondary care activity into primary care, also need to be carefully scrutinised in order to make sure that they do not harm patients (and that, ideally, they are actually of benefit to patients!). In accordance with the available evidence, it would seem quite reasonable for general practitioners to excise skin lesions or undertake endoscopies, provided that they have the training and facilities to do so and are appropriately accredited. However, primary care services must also be subject to the same quality-control and prospective audit procedures as would apply in the secondary care setting. In a study in North Thames of skin cancers excised by general practitioners, it was noted that there was a tendency towards incomplete excision of lesions and under-usage of histopathology services.[37]

Currently there is much enthusiasm for GPs undertaking the follow-up of cancer patients in remission. In the case of both breast cancer and colorectal cancer there are pressures within secondary care causing hospital trusts to seek to extricate themselves from some of the burden associated with long-term follow-up of such patients. Furthermore, randomised controlled trials in Italy (now with ten years of follow-up) have shown that less intensive breast cancer follow-up is not associated with adverse outcomes.[38]

Grunfeld and colleagues have undertaken a randomised controlled trial in Oxfordshire in which they compared follow-up by general practitioners with usual care from one of two hospital outpatient clinics. They found that GP care resulted in no increase in the time to diagnosis, no increase in anxiety and no deterioration in quality of life, as well as enhanced satisfaction and lower costs to patients and the health service.[39,40] However, when examining the applicability of these results, it is important to appreciate that the patients studied may have been significantly dissimilar from the patients who would be encountered in other settings. Unfortunately, no information was provided on important demographic factors such as ethnicity and social class. In addition, one-third of the patients who were invited to become involved in the trial chose not to participate, and these were generally the older women. The GPs who were involved in the study were given time to undergo a period of training, and received a detailed letter from the hospital together with an information package. In addition, it is important to note that the outcomes were relatively short term, and it is necessary to know the effect on longer-term outcomes such as mortality. Finally, there is a requirement for further research into the symptoms and signs of recurrence among the population of patients who are being followed up by general practitioners.

When the initial results of Grunfeld's study were first published in 1996, many health authorities were keen to take the initiative and to shift services into primary care. They adopted a somewhat selective interpretation of the available evidence, and the experience to date has indicated some resistance from primary care. Therefore, in moving matters forward there is a need for both more and better evidence, as well as seeking to ensure that the new service is a sensible and realistic alternative to current practice. There will also be a need to link any considerations related to cancer follow-up within primary care to issues relating to clinical capacity, clinical governance and possibly cancer accreditation. Work by Randev and colleagues (P Randev, personal communication) has demonstrated that primary care cancer services can be well supported and assured by a framework of standards developed and tested within primary care.

With the involvement of many general practitioners in the commissioning of care and the establishment of primary care clinical cancer leads, there is now an additional obligation on primary care professionals to ensure that the local oncology provision is of the best possible quality. Services need to be effective, efficient and delivered in an acceptable, accessible and equitable fashion. In recent years, important geographical variations in outcomes following treatment for breast or colorectal cancer have been highlighted, and the Calman–Hine developments have sought to address some of these problems.[2] In the future, primary care clinicians working with their public health and secondary care colleagues as members of primary care trusts and within cancer networks will have a particularly important role to play in ensuring equity and accessibility in relation to cancer care.[41] For most major cancers there is continuing evidence that patients from affluent areas have better survival rates than patients from deprived neighbourhoods.[42] However, there is an urgent need for a 'National Primary Care Advisory Group' to be formed in order to ensure that there is consistency across the UK. Differences in primary care cancer interest between primary care groupings could easily create further inequalities, and this is the very thing that the NHS Cancer Plan sets out to address.

Conclusion

In seeking both to improve cancer services and to involve primary care in such developments there is a requirement to consider extremely carefully what role primary care professionals should or could play in delivering better cancer care. The internal and external validity of all published evidence needs to be rigorously examined, and it is essential that there is a clear understanding of the capacity and commitment within primary care. The dictum espoused by Hippocrates of *primum non nocere* (first do no harm) is nowhere more appropriate than in the discussion of developments in primary care oncology, where the political and managerial imperatives are so powerful. As is well illustrated by the development of cancer referral guidance, if primary care clinicians do not take the initiative in determining the future direction for primary care oncology, then others certainly will.

References

1   Department of Health (2000) *The NHS Cancer Plan*. Department of Health, London.

2   Department of Health (1995) *A Policy Framework for Commissioning Cancer Services. A Report by the Expert Advisory Group on Cancer to the Chief Medical Officer of England and Wales*. Department of Health, London.

3   Nylenna M (1986) A survey of cancer patients in general practice. *Fam Pract.* **3**: 168–73.

4   Gorman DR, Mackinnon H, Storrie M *et al.* (2000) The general practice perspective on cancer services in Lothian. *Fam Pract.* **17**: 323–8.

5   McWhinney IR, Hoddinott SN, Bass MJ *et al.* (1990) Role of the family physician in the care of cancer patients. *Can Fam Physician.* **36**: 2183–6.

6   Hargarten SW, Roberts MJS and Anderson AJ (1992) Cancer presentation in the emergency department; a failure of primary care. *Am J Emerg Med.* **10**: 290–3.

7   Richards MA, Westcombe AM, Love SB *et al.* (1999) Influence of delay on survival in patients with breast cancer: a systematic review. *Lancet.* **353**: 1119–26.

8   Green S and Price J (1998) Complaints. *Pulse.* **4 April**: 63, 67.

9   Berrino F, Capocaccia R, Esteve J *et al.* (eds) (1999) *Survival for Cancer Patients in Europe: the Eurocare II Study*. International Agency for Research on Cancer, Lyons.

10 Roetzheim RG, Pal N, Gonzalez EC *et al.* (1999) The effects of physician supply on the early detection of colorectal cancer. *J Fam Pract.* **48**: 850–8.

11 Summerton N (1999) *Diagnosing Cancer in Primary Care*. Radcliffe Medical Press, Oxford.

12 Department of Health (1999) *Cancer Waiting Times: achieving the two-week target*. HSC 1999/205. Department of Health, London.

13 NHS Centre for Reviews and Dissemination (1994) *Effective Health Care. Implementing clinical practice guidelines*. University of York, York.

14 Liedekerken BMJ, Hoogendam A, Buntinx F *et al.* (1997) Prolonged cough and lung cancer: the need for more general practice research to inform clinical decision making. *Br J Gen Pract.* **47**: 505.

15 Bruntinx F and Wauters H (1997) The diagnostic value of macroscopic haematuria in diagnosing urological cancers: a meta-analysis. *Fam Pract.* **14**: 63–8.

16 Froom P, Froom J and Ribak J (1997) Asymptomatic microscopic haematuria – is investigation necessary? *J Clin Epidemiol.* **11**: 1197–200.

17 Muris JWM, Starmans R, Fijten GH *et al.* (1995) Non-acute abdominal complaints in general practice: diagnostic value of signs and symptoms. *Br J Gen Pract.* **45**: 313–16.

18 McWhinney IR (1962) The early diagnosis of cancer. *J Coll Gen Pract.* **5**: 404–14.

19 Starey CJH (1966) The diagnosis and treatment of cancer in a general practice. *J Coll Gen Pract.* **12**: 32–42.

20 Owen P (1995) Clinical practice and medical research: bridging the divide between the two cultures. *Br J Gen Pract.* **45**: 557–60.

21 Summerton N (2000) Diagnosis and general practice. *Br J Gen Pract.* **50**: 995–1000.

22 House of Commons Science and Technology Committee (2000) *Cancer Research: a fresh look.* The Stationery Office, London.

23 Vecchio TJ (1966) Predictive value of a single diagnostic test in unselected populations. *NEJM.* **274**: 1171–3.

24 McWhinney IR (1999) *The Martin Bass Lecture. Why are we doing so little clinical research?* University of Toronto, Toronto.

25 Pereira-Gray DJ (1966) The role of general practitioners in the early detection of malignant disease. *Trans Hunterian Soc.* **25**: 135–79.

26 Nylenna M (1986) Diagnosing cancer in general practice: from suspicion to certainty. *BMJ.* **293**: 314–17.

27 Olesen F (1988) Pattern of attendance at general practice in the years before the diagnosis of cervical cancer: a case–control study. *Scand J Prim Health Care.* **6**: 199–203.

28 Summerton N and Paes R (2000) The clinical assessment of patients with large bowel symptoms by general practitioners. *Eur J Gen Pract.* **6**: 43–7.

29 Chalabian J, Formenti S, Russell C *et al.* (1998) Comprehensive needs assessment of clinical breast evaluation skills of primary care residents. *Ann Surg Oncol.* **5**: 166–72.

30 Del Mar CB and Green AC (1995) Aid to diagnosis of melanoma in primary care. *BMJ.* **310**: 492–5.

31 Boyer KL, Ford MB, Judkins AF and Levin B (1999) *Primary Care Oncology.* WB Saunders Co., Philadelphia, PA.

32 Silvestri GA, Littenberg B and Colice GL (1995) The clinical evaluation for detecting metastatic lung cancer. A meta-analysis. *Am J Respir Crit Care Med.* **152**: 225–30.

33 Coeburgh JWW, Janssen-Heijnen MLG, Post PN and Razenberg PPA (1999) Serious comorbidity among unselected cancer patients newly diagnosed in the south-eastern part of the Netherlands in 1993–1996. *J Clin Epidemiol.* **52**: 1131–6.

34 Jones R, Pearson J, McGregor S *et al.* (1999) Cross-sectional survey of patients' satisfaction with information about cancer. *BMJ.* **319**: 1247–8.

35 Redelmeier DA, Tan SH and Booth GL (1998) The treatment of unrelated disorders in patients with chronic medical diseases. *NEJM.* **338**: 1516–20.

36 Yu GP, Ostroff JS, Zhang ZF *et al.* (1997) Smoking history and cancer patient survival: a hospital cancer registry study. *Cancer Detect Prev.* **21**: 497–509.

37 Khorshid SM, Pinney E and Newton-Bishop JA (1998) Melanoma excision by general practitioners in North-East Thames region, England. *Br J Dermatol.* **138**: 412–17.

38 Palli D, Russo A, Saieva C *et al.* (1999) Intensive vs. clinical follow-up after treatment for primary breast cancer: 10-year update of a randomised trial. *JAMA.* **281**: 1586.

39 Grunfeld E, Fitzpatrick R, Mant D *et al.* (1999) Comparison of breast cancer patient satisfaction with follow-up in primary care versus specialist care: result from a randomised controlled trial. *Br J Gen Pract.* **49**: 705–10.

40 Grunfeld E, Mant D, Yudkin P *et al.* (1996) Routine follow-up of breast cancer in primary care: a randomised trial. *BMJ.* **313**: 665–9.

41 Davey C, Austoker A and Macleod K (1999) *Reducing Inequalities in Breast Cancer: a guide for primary care.* Cancer Research Campaign, London.

42 Ozonoff D and Clapp R (1999) Cancer survival is no lottery. *Lancet.* **353**: 1379–80.

CHAPTER 9

Postgraduate medical education for modern cancer services

Rosemary Macdonald and Roger Taylor

Introduction

The purpose of postgraduate medical education must surely be to educate and train the doctors who are required by the NHS.

These doctors will receive postgraduate education to standards determined by the General Medical Council (undergraduate curriculum, preregistration house officer (PRHO) year) and the relevant Royal Colleges and Faculties (senior house officers (SHOs) and specialist registrars (SpRs)).

For the first time since the inception of the NHS, the medical profession and those responsible for medical education are being given explicit guidelines on the type of healthcare delivery that is required by patients.[1-3]

The New NHS: Modern, Dependable[1] set out the Government's basic concepts. The NHS Plan[2] particularised those concepts, and the NHS Cancer Plan[3] provides a blueprint for cancer care, with targets to be achieved by certain dates. This had been pre-dated by the Calman–Hine Report,[4] which set in motion structural and organisational changes to lay the foundations for the implementation of the NHS Cancer Plan.[3]

Many governmental publications talk about a 'modern service' or 'modernising services'. It is important to clarify the meaning of the terms 'modern' and 'modernising'. The Oxford English Dictionary defines 'modern' as 'new; not existing before', but in middle English (i.e. Chaucer), 'modern' means 'to take a fresh look'.

This is precisely what is happening to cancer services – 'a fresh look' at the organisation and provision of care. Therefore it behoves those who are responsible for medical education to take a 'fresh look' at the education and

---

Box 9.1:   *Duties of a Doctor: Good Medical Practice* (General Medical Council, 1995)

Good medical practice	The main parts of *Good Medical Practice* set out below:
Good clinical care	• practise good standards of clinical care • make sure that patients are not put at unnecessary risk • work within the limits of their professional competence.
Maintaining good medical practice	Doctors must: • keep their knowledge and skills up to date • regularly take part in educational activities that develop their skills • try to act on what is said during appraisals.
Relationships with patients	Doctors must: • make the care of their patients their first concern • treat every patient politely and considerately • respect patients' dignity and privacy • listen to patients and respect their views • give information to patients in a form that they can understand • respect patients' right to be fully involved in decisions about their treatment.
Working with colleagues	Doctors must work effectively with their medical and non-medical colleagues as well as other healthcare professionals. Co-operation, trust and flexibility are essential to good patient care.
Teaching and training	Doctors with special teaching responsibilities must: • develop the skills, attitudes and practices of a competent teacher • be honest and objective when they are assessing the performance of someone they have trained.
Honesty and integrity	Doctors must: • be honest and trustworthy • respect and protect confidential information • make sure that their personal beliefs do not interfere with patients' care • act quickly to protect their patients from any risk • not abuse their position.
Health	If a doctor has a serious condition that could affect their performance, or could be passed on to patients, they must seek and follow advice from an appropriate colleague.

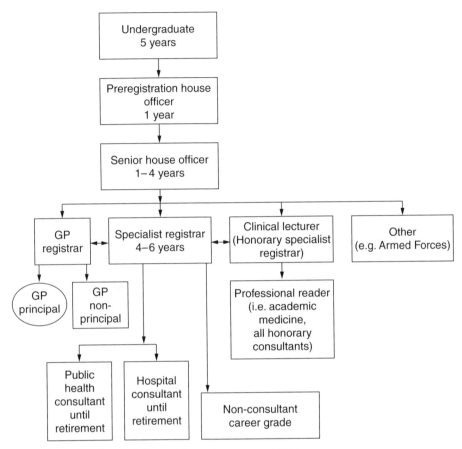

Note: Occasionally specialist registrars change specialties.
Note: Occasionally consultants and GP principals diversify within their career grade posts.

Figure 9.1: Doctor's career pathway.

training of doctors. A basic tenet is that the product should exhibit performance that is compliant with *Good Medical Practice*[5] (*see* Box 9.1) and have the knowledge, skills and attitudes to be a competent, caring doctor.

How has medical education responded to the demands? Figure 9.1 shows a doctor's career pathway and the average duration of each stage.

Selection of medical students

The traditional beer-swilling, rugby-playing, male middle-class student from a public school has yielded to a rich diversity of students that reflects our population (i.e. women, ethnic minorities, state-educated students, non-graduate parents, etc.). The Higher Education Funding Council has approved bids from medical schools to expand their numbers. New medical schools are also being developed. Guidelines encouraged bids to demonstrate a commitment to 'wider access' (i.e. to offer undergraduate medical education to many more mature students and graduates with non-science degrees). Access and foundation courses will be provided for such entrants, often using the facilities of the Open University. Thus the profile of our medical student population will change further.[6] We hope that the profile of our undergraduates will reflect that of our patients and thus enhance the doctor–patient relationship. Academic medicine and research (both basic and applied) will not be forgotten.

Undergraduate medical education and the pre-registration house officer year

The General Medical Council anticipated many of these requirements almost a decade ago. *Tomorrow's Doctors*[7] provides details of the changes in the undergraduate curriculum which almost all medical schools have implemented. *The New Doctor*[8] gave guidance to those responsible for the preregistration house officer year. Points of relevance to cancer services are listed in Boxes 9.2 and 9.3.

Box 9.2: *Tomorrow's Doctors*: recommendations on undergraduate medical education that are pertinent to cancer srvices (General Medical Council, 1993)

Core curriculum (*mandatory*)	To ensure essential knowledge and skills; systems teaching (e.g. heart disease). Vertical/ horizontal integration (e.g. physiology, biochemistry, diagnosis, therapy, rehabilitation and epidemiology – all focused on specific disease entities)
Special study modules (*menu of topics available*)	Students study the topic in depth; provides insights into scientific methods, research, etc., and the totality of a disease
Goals	Knowledge and understanding of disease prevention; health promotion; acquisition of basic clinical skills; development of attitudes (i.e. good medical practice)

Curriculum themes	Clinical methods; practical skills; patient care; communication skills; human biology; human disease; man in society; public health

Undergraduate medical education is now more learner centred, more problem orientated with much small group work (embryonic teams), less reliant on didactic teaching, and capitalises on natural intellectual curiosity.

Box 9.3: *The New Doctor*: recommendations on general clinical training that are pertinent to cancer services (General Medical Council, 1992)

The philosophy	*Good Medical Practice* should underpin the preregistration house officer year
Communication skills	Practice in a *multicultural society; prevention* of illness; promotion of health
Ethical and legal aspects of medical practice	
Teamwork and collective responsibility	
Evidence-based medicine	Informatics
Psychological and social factors in illness	Pain relief; care of the dying; *care of the bereaved*
Self-education and professional development	

'The early years': senior house officer years[9]

Although some sixth-formers enter medical school with preconceived career objectives (e.g. 'I want to be a surgeon'), most formulate realistic plans during the PRHO year. The senior house officer grade enables the doctor to capitalise upon and extend his or her knowledge and clinical skills acquired during the PRHO year. Many choose broad-based senior house officer rotations that provide experience in the 'generality' of medical or surgical specialties. Basic

---

Box 9.4: *The Early Years*: recommendations on senior house officer
training that are pertinent to cancer services (General Medical
Council, 2000)

Further	develop generic medical knowledge and skills, as well as appropriate professional attitudes.
Begin	to develop specialty-specific knowledge and skills.
Further	develop *personal transferable skills* (e.g. communication, teamworking).
Foster	an interest in and knowledge of research.
Enhance	appreciation of evidence-based practice and clinical effectiveness.
Refine	understanding of management issues and clinical audit.

---

postgraduate examinations have to be passed during this time in order to gain entry to the specialist registrar grade. Box 9.4 lists the recommendations for that grade that are relevant to cancer care.

Training for senior house officers in oncology

A prerequisite for entry to either a clinical or medical oncology (radiotherapy and chemotherapy, respectively) specialist registrar training scheme is general medical experience and passing of the MRCP examination (Membership of the Royal College of Physicians). The majority of oncology departments can provide valuable experience for trainees who are preparing for the MRCP and wish to pursue a career in any of the oncological or associated specialties, such as palliative care or haematology. A recent survey of senior house officer posts in clinical oncology[10] showed that 50% of these posts were part of a fixed medical rotation.

Traditionally, the main role of senior house officers in clinical and medical oncology has been 'ward work' (i.e. supervision of the care of patients who have been admitted for radiotherapy or chemotherapy). They also manage side-effects and elements of palliative care. As a consequence, the view of oncology from the perspective of a ward-based senior house officer can become skewed. They need to experience the full therapeutic range and see successes. Good education and training of this grade with adequate assessment may assist recruitment.[10]

Specialist registrar years

This is the grade between senior house officer and consultant. Education and training during this grade enables the doctor to acquire the Certificate of Completion of Specialist Training (CCST). Specialist registrars progress through planned rotations designed to give them the knowledge, skills and attitudes to be specialists or consultants. Progression through this grade is dependent on satisfactory appraisals and annual assessments. The first and final assessments are the most important – the former should 'weed out' those who are unsuitable for the specialty, and the latter identifies that the trainee is *competent* to be an independently practising consultant, taking responsibility for training others. Trainees in clinical oncology also have to pass the national Fellow of the Royal College of Radiologists (FRCR) examinations.

Overview

Virtually every specialty will participate in the delivery of cancer services, from the most obvious, such as general practitioners, surgeons and clinical and medical oncologists, to occupational health physicians and public health consultants.

Educating doctors to deliver cancer care requires generic clinical and non-clinical skills to which are added specialty-specific clinical and non-clinical skills, never losing the basic tenets of *Good Medical Practice*.[5]

Hopefully, the foundation and incremental training of the future cancer specialist can be understood. Each training grade expands on the clinical and non-clinical skills acquired. Finally, the specialist or consultant emerges able to be responsible for his or her self-directed lifelong learning through continuing professional education. This is now an important cancer centre function which could provide a continuum of education linking postgraduate education with consultant professional and personal development.

Ensuring competence: ensuring valid assessment

Patients and carers want competent caring doctors, but what is competence in the context of the totality of patient care?

Competence was ranked first of nine core values to guide the medical profession into the twenty-first century.[11]

But what is competence in relation to medical practice? Calman[12] stated that 'the exact definition of competence requires further work, but it is at the heart of ensuring that practising doctors in all specialties have the *appropriate skills and attributes*'.

A definition remains elusive. The 'attributes of the independent practitioner' and 'good medical practice'[5] have been identified, yet specifying competence is the cornerstone of valid assessment along the whole continuum of undergraduate, postgraduate and continuing medical education.

Competence is usually perceived in one of two ways – first, the ability to perform discrete tasks (i.e. clinical skills), and secondly, the ability to transfer underlying cognitive abilities such as decision making and problem solving to new situations.

Safe effective patient care requires an amalgamation of knowledge, skills *and* attitudes. Therefore it is more than mere competence.[13] 'Integrated competence' draws together all of these constituent strands and encapsulates the whole of a doctor's performance. Thus priority might at times be given to the non-clinical skills implicit within the doctor's role as team leader or team member. Integrated competence supplements the knowledge requirements hitherto demanded by the General Medical Council and Royal Colleges in a way which captures the professional's and patients' concepts of being a good doctor (i.e. good medical practice).[5]

Individual competencies

A qualitative study conducted in the Yorkshire Deanery[14] endeavoured to identify the 'core competencies' of senior house officers. Ready consensus was obtained and the work has now been extended to other grades to form a basis for assessment.

The core competencies are as follows:

- *knowledge:* all doctors must have an adequate knowledge of their subject
- *skills:* practical and psychomotor skills
- *attitudes/attributes:* these terms tend to be used synonymously, but are subtly different; attitudes constitute a way of behaving, whereas attributes are individual qualities and characteristics. Attitudes are more difficult but not impossible to modify.

Non-clinical skills are the most difficult to assess. The study subdivided these further as follows:

- *professional and personal development:* this encompasses career planning, lifelong learning, and maturation both as an individual and as a doctor

- *supervisory skills:* progress of the profession depends on doctors' ability to per-form their *supervisory* role effectively (e.g. trainees are expected to teach, supervise and support more junior medical trainees and other professionals who are contributing to patient care). At times consultants will learn from trainees – education and training are mutual processes. Both should learn from patients
- *managerial skills:* this composite describes the increasingly verbalised roles that are required to deliver successful patient care (e.g. time management, prioritisation, communication, assertiveness, presentation skills, team mem-bership and leadership). For each specialty there are *core* and *specialty-specific* managerial roles.

All of the Royal Colleges, including the Royal College of Physicians (for medical oncologists) and the Royal College of Radiologists (for clinical oncologists), are developing procedures for defining levels of competence that the trainee must have acquired at defined stages in specialist registrar training, particu-larly prior to the award of a CCST. These levels need to be defined across a range of competencies, and defined by a series of 'descriptors'. The attainment of these levels will be validated by consultant trainers. Descriptors need to be as precise as possible so that they can be used to define national standards for competence. *See* Appendix to this chapter.

Team competencies

Patient care, particularly cancer care, is delivered by a team. Implementation of the Calman–Hine Report[4] has resulted in the evolution of many multidisciplin-ary and multiprofessional teams for the management of patients in cancer units and centres. A dysfunctional team will not provide good care.

Currently, a project in the Yorkshire Deanery[15] is aiming to identify the core competencies of clinical teams in three priority healthcare areas (coronary heart disease, old age psychiatry and cancer care).

The concept of patient care provided by a team is not straightforward. Many team members will belong to several teams and will be leaders in their own fields. Also, as each individual patient is a focus of team activities, continuous reconstruction of the team may be necessary. At least the English cricket team have only one focus (to win) and each has a well-defined role, but Brearley[16] still found it necessary to treat his team members as individuals, and occasion-ally to give priority to the needs of the individual.

Although these are early days, the project is beginning to define *units* and *ele-ments* of competence, as follows:

- establishing and maintaining effective relationships with 'clients' (i.e. establishing, maintaining and facilitating relationships with patients and all of their carers)
- contributing effectively to discussions and decisions about patient management (e.g. sharing information to inform the decision-making process)
- contributing towards the development of effective team delivery:
    (i)   understanding the range of roles within the team
    (ii) contributing to the development of an effective team ethos and vision
    (iii) supporting the development of other team members
- contributing to the establishment and maintenance of effective working relationships:
    (i)   responding flexibly to situations
    (ii) resolving conflicts constructively
    (iii) maintaining personal stability under pressure
- contributing to quality improvement in patient care:
    (i)   reviewing team performance to improve delivery
    (ii) striving to improve individual performance.

Once agreement has been reached about the units and elements of competence, then a framework for team assessment will follow.

This is in broad agreement with Brealey's 'lessons' – that is, 'good teams consist of groups of strongly characterised individuals and the art of leading such a team is *not* to suppress individuality but to harness it to achieve the teams goals'[16] – all very relevant to cancer teams.

Interprofessional, multiprofessional education and teamworking

The identification of core competencies of teams will enable not only team assessment but also team training and education. The NHS Plan[3] is committed to joint training for all healthcare professionals in non-clinical generic skills (e.g. communication).

In order to provide good cancer care, team education and training need to be disease focused. It is envisaged that substitution will take place, and this is very challenging for both the medical and non-medical 'tribes', particularly as cognate abilities may vary widely. Finch[17] eloquently summarises interprofessional education and teamworking as follows: 'The organisational challenges would be considerable – *but the gains could be enormous*'. This is particularly so for cancer patients.

Clinical and medical oncology training for modern cancer services

The specialties of clinical and medical oncology have evolved from different backgrounds. Historically, clinical oncologists were based in oncology centres and provided a 'visiting radiotherapy' and sometimes a chemotherapy service to district general hospitals. They are linked to radiologists by the common use of ionising radiation, and training and service standards are monitored by the Royal College of Radiologists. The emphasis was on delivery of a regional service, and it generally involved a high workload. Most clinical oncologists supervise the prescription and administration of both radiotherapy and chemotherapy, and have developed site-specialised expertise. Many of them also undertake clinical research.

Medical oncology is a relatively new specialty which developed from general medicine and clinical haematology. Consultants tend to practise in oncology centres. Posts are frequently academic and have often been funded by cancer charities. In most units there is a strong emphasis on laboratory and developmental clinical research. Training and service issues are monitored by the Royal College of Physicians.

Training in the two specialties has reflected these differing backgrounds.[18] The basis of training for clinical oncologists has been a broad-based structured training leading to the FRCR examination. Medical oncology training often includes the acquisition of research skills leading to a higher degree, but with no formal examination beyond the MRCP.

However, the boundaries between the two disciplines have recently become more blurred, and there is increasing use of either sequential or concurrent chemotherapy and radiotherapy. In many cancer centres, clinical and medical oncologists are working together in a multidisciplinary environment based on clinical research.

The most important factor which is 'driving' changes in the organisation of cancer services in cancer units (district general hospitals) is the implementation of the Calman–Hine Report.[4] Management of common cancers is based on multidisciplinary and multiprofessional teams. There is no need to move from a busy 'visiting radiotherapy and chemotherapy' service to the provision of comprehensive non-surgical oncology expertise, with clinical and/or medical oncologists providing site-specialised input to cancer units. The administration of chemotherapy for common cancers needs to be supervised in the cancer unit, whereas patients who require radiotherapy need to travel to the cancer centre. Clinical oncology training is broad-based, validated by a national examination, and can provide the necessary training for an oncologist to be the initial adviser for the patient with cancer. He or she can then refer the patient to another oncologist if different site-specialist expertise is required, but a clinical oncologist must spend a significant amount of time in the cancer centre in order to supervise the planning and administration of chemotherapy.

Medical oncology training has been traditionally more focused, without a national examination. Most medical oncologists train in specialised academic centres, which may not prepare them to supervise the 'holistic care' of the patient, including palliative care services, in a cancer unit. There is currently considerable discussion about the optimum method for providing 'resident' oncology services in a cancer unit. In some cancer units in the UK, resident medical oncologists provide 'holistic' cancer care. In others this care is provided by several clinical oncologists, each contributing a degree of site-specialised expertise and spending significant amounts of time in the cancer unit. The question of how to provide the best service for patients in cancer units remains controversial and unresolved.

Common ('core') training for clinical and medical oncologists

Much of the knowledge, many of the skills and certainly the attitudes that need to be acquired during specialist registrar training are common to clinical and medical oncologists. Knowledge of the basic oncological sciences underpins sound clinical practice. All oncologists require excellent communication skills in relating both to patients and their families and to medical and non-medical colleagues. They also need to acquire skills in the management of palliative care. Other generic skills include teamworking, leadership and time management. They need to learn about hospital and NHS management, including the principles of implementation of clinical governance, resource management and cost-effectiveness and information technology.

The majority of medical and clinical oncology trainees would like more joint training,[19] resulting in the ability to treat many common cancers with radiotherapy and chemotherapy. Most clinical oncologists do not wish to be radiotherapists (i.e. to prescribe only radiotherapy). Medical oncologists could easily be trained to prescribe routine protocol-based radiotherapy, particularly if they were aided by the inclusion of therapeutic radiographers and medical physicists within the cancer centre multiprofessional teams. If clinical and medical oncology training commenced with the 'core' elements, then during the latter stages of training specialist registrars could diversify mainly into either medical or clinical oncology and also site specialise. A few oncologists in cancer centres would care mainly for the rare cancers and also provide and scientifically assess innovative therapies before the implementation of their widespread use.

Although treatments and rare cancers require highly specialised individuals, more joint clinical and medical oncology training will enhance the management of patients with common and intermediate-frequency cancers.

Whatever the background of the oncologist, they will need sufficient knowledge of the breadth of oncology to act as the 'initial adviser' to the patient with cancer. They will then organise treatment or (more frequently) refer the patient to an appropriate colleague in the team with the necessary expertise.

The Joint Collegiate Council for Oncology (JCCO) is a body whose function is to oversee service and training issues that are common to clinical and medical oncology. The JCCO reports to the respective colleges (the Royal College of Physicians for medical oncologists and the Royal College of Radiologists for clinical oncologists), and has established an education committee which is in the process of designing a programme for 'core training' in clinical and medical oncology. This will include the knowledge and clinical experience of all oncologists.

Both specialties must 'grasp the nettle' of joint training if cancer services are to be modernised. The talents of *all* the members of the cancer care team *must* be utilised.

Training surgical oncologists

Postgraduate educational training for surgeons consists of six years at the specialist registrar grade. During years five and six, trainees subspecialise (e.g. in breast and endocrine, colorectal, gastro-oesophageal or hepatobiliary cancers, etc.). Those who envisage a career as a surgical oncologist may also take a year 'out of programme' to train in a highly specialised unit either in the UK or overseas. This not only enhances their surgical skills, but also assists their total personal and professional development as a surgical oncologist.

Those who are responsible for education and training would wish for more of our potential surgical oncologists to have *ad personam* programmes that include time in oncological disciplines as well as some community experience. Trainees emerge with a CCST in general surgery with a subspecialty interest and then apply for relevant posts at consultant level.

Gynaecological surgical oncology training is well developed under the auspices of the Royal College of Obstetricians and Gynaecologists. These are recognised training programmes with numbered funded posts. Specialist registrars in obstetrics and gynaecology compete for these 'subspecialty training posts' and embark upon a 2 to 4-year training programme, depending on previous experience, in which they are virtually supernumerary and training can be almost *ad personam*. This programme includes one year in general gynaecological oncology and one year in research, all in a cancer centre. The programme is modular and includes time in a hospice, and attachments to Macmillan nurses, pain therapists, etc. This 'subspecialty training programme' is a model which other specialties could well emulate. Trainees emerge with a CCST in obstetrics and gynaecology, with a subspecialty interest.

Planning the workforce

The NHS Cancer Plan[3] states that by the year 2006 there will be an extra 1000 cancer specialists. There will also be investment in the training and development of other healthcare professionals and non-health professionals (e.g. social workers) whose role is crucial to improving outcomes.

The term 'cancer specialist' embraces many different specialties. Some, such as clinical oncologists (prescribing radiotherapy and chemotherapy) and medical oncologists (providing general medical care and prescribing chemotherapy) work exclusively with cancer patients. Other specialists, such as palliative care physicians, pathologists, radiologists, surgeons, clinical haematologists, respiratory physicians, anaesthetists, etc., will care for patients with other diseases. However, in cancer centres some will 'specialise', thereby gaining much expertise which should be harnessed to educate and train tomorrow's cancer specialists.

Health authorities and PCTs in partnership with trusts need to identify funding to plan the development of more consultant posts linked to the expected output of CCST holders. Training capacity is often limited because there are not enough consultants to undertake the training. Moreover, trainees require 'all-round' experience and should rotate through both cancer units and cancer centres as well as attending peripheral clinics.

If possible, those trainees from non-mainline cancer specialties (e.g. general surgery) should spend a little time observing other specialties (e.g. radiotherapy planning sessions, hospice work, etc.). The ultimate aim must be to produce consultants with an 'all-round' knowledge of the disease and how it affects not only patients but also families and communities. Cross-referrals should be relevant.

Strategic Health Authorities and Postgraduate Deans[20] will need to work very closely together, with the new Chief Executives of Workforce Confederations having an important co-ordinating role. Royal Colleges will continue to advise and ensure that training standards are met. Trust Medical Directors and Chief Executives must also ensure the development of robust cancer teams. Radical thinking and breaking down of barriers are necessary.

An important challenge is to identify the 'mix' of oncologists required by the NHS of the twenty-first century. In order to meet the expectations of the ageing population there needs to be continued expansion of cancer services for the foreseeable future. The needs of the population must be identified in order to guide trainees towards relevant specialties and subspecialty interests (e.g. it is wasteful to permit the training of too many gynaecological oncologists or to develop surgeons with a service/training mismatch of subspecialty interests). Most thoracic surgical trainees wish to be cardiac surgeons. Some of them must be encouraged to become lung cancer surgeons, but how many?

Our 'service needs' appraisal and manpower planning are not yet sufficiently sophisticated, but must become so. The present moulds of clinical and medical oncology require reassessment. Since support specialties such as histopathology, haematology and diagnostic radiology are crucial to outcomes, planning and funding for their trainees must not be forgotten. Finally, palliative medicine and pain therapy should be included in the 'training to treat cancer' blueprint.

Conclusion

Medical education and training to treat cancer have developed rapidly during the last decade. The next challenge is to bring more care into the community and home.

References

1   NHS Executive. (1998) *The New NHS: modern, dependable. A national framework for assessing performance*. NHS Executive, Leeds.

2   Department of Health (2000) *The NHS Plan: a plan for investment, a plan for reform*. Department of Health, London.

3   NHS Executive (2000) *The NHS Career Plan: a plan for investment, a plan for return*. NHS Executive, Leeds.

4   Department of Health (1995) *A Policy Framework for Commissioning Cancer Services; a Report by the Expert Advisory Group on Cancer to the Chief Medical Officers of England and Wales*. Department of Health, London.

5   General Medical Council (1995) *Duties of a Doctor: good medical practice*. General Medical Council, London.

6   Angel C and Johnson A (2000) Broadening access to undergraduate medical education. *BMJ*. **321**: 1136–8.

7 General Medical Council (1993) *Tomorrow's Doctors. Recommendations on undergraduate medical education.* General Medical Council, London.

8 General Medical Council (1997) *The New Doctor. Recommendations on general clinical training.* General Medical Council, London.

9 General Medical Council (1998) *The Early Years. Recommendations on senior house officer training.* General Medical Council, London.

10 Taylor RE and Macdonald R (2000) Education and training of senior house officers in clinical oncology departments. *Clin Oncol.* **12**: 42–7.

11 British Medical Association (1995) *Core Values for the Medical Profession in the Twenty-first Century.* Health Policy and Economic Research Unit, London.

12 Calman K (1996) Departmental news from the Chief Medical Officer. *Health Trends.* **28**: 1–2.

13 Hager P and Gonczi A (1996) What is competence? *Med Teacher.* **18**: 15–18.

14 Ilott I and Allen M (1996) *Identification of Core Competencies of Senior House Officers as Prerequisites for Higher Specialty Training.* Department for Education and Employment and Department of Health, London.

15 Pickering C and Allen M (2000) *Project on Core Competencies of Clinical Teams.* Jointly funded by the West Yorkshire Consortium and Yorkshire Deanery, Leeds.

16 Brearley M (2000) Teams: lessons from the world of sport. Based on a presentation from the Millennium Festival of Medicine. *BMJ.* **321**: 1141–3.

17 Finch J (2000) Interprofessional education and teamworking: a view from the education providers. *BMJ.* **321**: 1138–40.

18 Dodwell D, Sebag-Montefiore D, Collinson M and Selby P (1999) Delivery of non-surgical oncology care. *Hosp Med.* **60**: 664–7.

19 Gerrard G, Short S, Hatton M *et al.* (1998) The future of oncology training: from the trainee's perspective. *Clin Oncol.* **10**: 84–91.

20 Department of Health (2000) *A Health Service of All the Talents: developing the NHS workforce.* Department of Health, London.

Appendix

JOINT COMMITTEE ON HIGHER SURGICAL TRAINING
TRAINEE ASSESSMENT FORM

This is an official document. The original is the property of the JCHST. For the annual assessment process the JCHST office will make the forms available, on request, to the Programme Directors who will supervise their completion by the appropriate trainer(s). The forms will be signed upon completion, by the trainer(s) and the trainee before the original copy is returned to the JCHST office at the Royal College of Surgeons of England. Photocopies of the forms should be passed to the **Programme Director, the Trainer(s), Regional Postgraduate Dean and the Intercollegiate Board if appropriate only**. Please ensure that the details in the box below are completed. **This form will be returned if incomplete, resulting in a delay for process**.

TRAINEE:	NTN/VTN/FTN OR LAT:
SPECIALITY:	YEAR: 6mths 1 2 3 4 5 6
ROTATION:	HOSPITAL:
PERIOD COVERING FROM:	TO:

CRITERIA	POOR	DEFICIENT	SATISFACTION (the majority of trainees)	GOOD	EXCELLENT	COMMENTS
A. Clinical skills						
History taking						
Physical exam						
Investigations						
Diagnosis						
Judgement						
Operative skill						
Aftercare						
B. Knowledge						
Basic science						
Clinical						
C. Postgraduate activities						
Teaching						
Lecturing style						
Case presentation						
Presentations						
Publications						
Research ability and audit						

CRITERIA	POOR	DEFICIENT	SATISFACTION (the majority of trainees)	GOOD	EXCELLENT	COMMENTS
D. Attitudes						
Reliability						
Self-motivation						
Leadership						
Administration						
Relationships with:						
a) Colleagues						
b) Patients						
c) Other staff						

TRAINER'S PEN PICTURE:

_____

_____

_____

_____

_____

_____

_____

_____

_____

_____

_____

TRAINER'S SIGNATURE(S): _____ /_____   DATE: _____
and NAME in block capitals
  _____ /_____

  _____ /_____

  _____ /_____

TRAINEE SIGNATURE: _____ /_____   DATE: _____

SIGNATURE OF THE TRAINEE INDICATES THAT HE/SHE HAS SEEN THE ASSESSMENT FORM, NOT THAT HE/SHE AGREES WITH ITS CONTENT. Trainees who disagree with the contents of this report may appeal in the first instance to the appropriate Specialist Advisory Committee and thence to the JCHST.

NOTES TO ACCOMPANY JCHST TRAINEE ASSESSMENT FORM

1.   The Assessment Form is CONFIDENTIAL once completed, and must be handled accordingly.

2.   The following guidelines are for trainers completing the form.

    a.   Complete as fully as possible the trainee details in the top box, circling the appropriate year of assessment.

    b.   Where more than one trainer is involved with the trainee, a consensus opinion should be expressed on the form, which should be signed by all trainers.

    c.   Complete the main assessment by placing an 'X' in one box only against each criterion. The comments box is available for additional comment if desired. The following guidelines are to be used when grading criteria. (SACs would expect most trainees to be graded SATISFACTORY if their training is progressing to a standard which would see them being recommended for the CCST.)

THE FORM WILL BE RETURNED IF INCOMPLETE.

	POOR/DEFICIENT	SATISFACTORY	GOOD/EXCELLENT
A. Clinical skills			
History taking	Incomplete. Inaccurate. Poorly recorded.	Usually complete, orderly and systematic.	Precise, perceptive, 'can spot the rarity'.
Physical exam	Lacks basic skills. Relies unnecessarily on investigations.	Can elicit correct signs. Recognises most significant findings.	Thorough, accurate. Knows and elicits specialist signs.
Investigations	Inappropriate, random. Unnecessarily expensive. Inability to interpret tests.	Usually appropriate. Good knowledge on interpreting tests (e.g. can read X-ray reliably).	Almost always appropriate in relation to differential diagnosis. Excellent at interpretation.
Diagnosis	Fails to interpret and synthesise symptoms, signs and investigations.	Complete clinician. Good knowledge with an orderly logical approach to differential diagnosis.	Outstanding diagnostician. Excellent clinical memory.
Judgement	Unreliable. Fails to grasp significance of findings or take appropriate action. Under- or over-reacts to emergencies.	Reliable. Competent under pressure. Asks for advice appropriately.	Outstanding clinician who is aware of his/her limits.
Operative skill (including endoscopy)	Clumsy, rough with tissues. Totally lacking in self-confidence technically.	Competent. Handles tissues well. Reliable endoscopist.	A master technician in both open and endoscopic surgery.
Aftercare	Uninterested. Fails to notice complications and act appropriately.	Conscientious. Good awareness for complications. Reliable in outpatients.	Excellent on wards. Notices problems early. Outstanding in follow-up outpatients.

B. Knowledge			
Basic science	Uninterested, does not read the literature. Fails to apply basic science knowledge to clinical problems.	Adequate fund of knowledge, and relates this satisfactorily to patient care.	Outstanding knowledge and understanding of the basic science of the speciality. Widely read.
Clinical	Poorly read. Lacks appropriate knowledge to construct a differential diagnosis. Fails to learn from experience.	Satisfactory knowledge for dealing with the common disorders. May fail to 'spot the rarity', but learns from experience.	Outstanding knowledge. Can be relied on to 'spot the rarity'. Widely read.

	POOR/DEFICIENT	SATISFACTORY	GOOD/EXCELLENT
C. Postgraduate activities			
Teaching	Uninterested and avoids teaching. Contributes little to the education of students or trainees in the grades below (e.g. SHOs).	Competent and conscientious in teaching others.	Excellent enthusiastic teacher. Can inspire.
Lecturing style	Avoids if possible. Poor style, poorly delivered, boring.	Reasonably well delivered. Competent but lacking 'spark'.	Excellent delivery. Dynamic. Logical and clear. Can 'hold' an audience.
Case presentation	Poor on history, signs, diagnosis and discussion.	Competent. History and signs correct. Good deductions.	Excellent presentation and discussion.
Presentations	No interest in giving papers. When has to, does it badly. Fails to get across a message.	Keen to give presentations which are well illustrated and well delivered.	Fully researched. Original ideas. Answers questions lucidly.
Publications	Shows no interest. Devoid of ideas. No grasp of English.	Keen, tries hard but lacking originality. Reasonable grasp of English.	An excellent CV. Many original ideas which are translated into published articles.
Research ability and audit	Has neither inclination nor ideas. Unable to carry out 'directed' projects. Not interested in audit.	Keen to do research and/or audit but needs considerable direction. Reasonable grasp of statistics and research methods.	Flair for original research with ability to carry out research independently. Utilises effective research methods.

	POOR/DEFICIENT	SATISFACTORY	GOOD/EXCELLENT
D. Attitudes			
Reliability	Unreliable, scatterbrained. Forgets to do things to the possible detriment of patients.	Dependable. Does not need reminding. Conscientious in patient care.	Highly conscientious. Anticipates problems.
Self-motivation	No inclination to organise work. Needs to be 'pushed' constantly.	Able to organise working routine without supervision. Looks for opportunities to learn.	Constantly pro-active, always prepared to accept additional opportunities to advance.
Leadership	Very limited. 'Switches people off'. Colleagues and other staff confused by his/her instructions.	Competent but lacks inspiration. Gives clear instructions.	Outstanding team leader with exceptional ability to motivate others.
Administration	Cannot be bothered. Always behind with letters and summaries. 'In a permanent muddle'.	Conscientious. Can be confidently left to deal with letters, summaries, waiting-lists, etc.	Excellent at routine administration. Has a good grasp of hospital management and politics.
Relationships with:			
a. Colleagues	Fails to get on with seniors, contemporaries or juniors. May even undermine them. Refuses to help out.	Good rapport with colleagues. Usually willing to help in a crisis. Trusted, easy to work with.	Always willing to help even if personally inconvenient. Able to defuse problems in the surgical team. 'An excellent colleague'.
b. Patients	Increases patients' anxieties. Rude. Patients do not want him/her as their doctor. Bad listener and communicator.	Sound, caring attitude. Can allay patients' fears. Takes time. Listens well, explains well. Trusted by the patient.	Inspires confidence. Establishes excellent rapport. Excellent communicator. Patients delighted to be looked after by him/her.
c. Other staff	Treats them with disdain. Generates as opposed to solving problems. Rude.	Sound and professional yet approachable. Treats others with respect and is respected in return.	Inspires enthusiasm. Exceptional communication skills.

3. Pen picture

Please summarise the trainee's character and overall performance, drawing attention to any outstanding features or alternatively ways in which the trainee failed to meet your expectations during this rotation. Do you foresee any specific difficulties/gaps in training that the trainee will have in completing his/her training?

CHAPTER 10

What cancer patients need

Mitzi Blennerhassett

Introduction

The extensive shortfalls in cancer services recognised in the NHS Plan[1] modernisation programme were later detailed by the NHS Cancer Plan,[2] which sets
out radical reform backed by cancer service standards and performance indicators along with action target dates. However, perhaps key to the Plan's reforms
is its claim to 'put the patient at the centre of cancer care'. Undoubtedly, the
quality of future commitment to user involvement at all levels will be seen by
patients and carers as crucial to the Plan's success.

   This chapter attempts to show why such reform is necessary, and discusses
the following:

- access and investigations
- consent
- treatment
- pain relief and palliative care
- allied humanitarian issues
- communication and information
- support
- accommodation and environment
- transport
- postcode prescribing, ageism and other inequalities
- the role of patient organisations in promoting change and monitoring performance.

Listening to other cancer patients in support groups and at national confer-
ences provides valuable insights into cancer service deficiences in this country – so much so wrong, yet until recently few people seemed to be willing or
able to speak out about the 'hidden' side of cancer care. Essentially, we need
co-ordinated cancer services which match the *best* of those in the developed

world, and efficient 'fast-track' systems for accessing them. However, equally important is our need to be treated with humanity.[3]

Access and investigations

Too-late referrals' have been commonplace, with many people presenting with symptoms to their general practitioner (GP) repeatedly for as long as two years before being referred to a consultant. Bowel cancer has been misdiagnosed as 'haemorrhoids', 'irritable bowel syndrome' or even 'arthritis', breast cancer has been misdiagnosed as 'benign fibroadenomas' or 'cysts', and ovarian cancer as 'diverticulitis'. Invariably, cancer has seemed to be last on the list of possibilities. Referral delays are too easily attributable to 'patient delay'.

It is argued that if every woman with a breast problem was seen within two weeks, clinics would be swamped with inappropriate referrals. Conversely, should women have to depend on getting an 'urgent' GP referral when even triple assessment is not always definitive? GPs may not read guidelines,[4] and local protocols may accommodate current levels of trust services by demanding less stringent criteria than national ones, so inviting fewer 'urgent' referrals. 'Of those waiting 12 weeks or more, "only" one in a hundred will turn out to have breast cancer' (Trust Executive). Would there be such complacency if these percentages applied to vaccination-damaged children? Waiting for investigations and results can initiate a cycle of decline, leaving patients less fit to undergo treatment.

> My medical notes state simply, 'There was a 5-month delay in her accessing treatment'. Despite immediately visiting my GP with obvious indicators, including my age and a discrete breast lump in the upper outer quadrant, my eventual referral was arranged only with difficulty, via the cytology clinic. At the same breast clinic a distracted woman paced the floor, having cried every night for 8 weeks.

We need:

- cancer training to offer GPs the support they deserve
- the 'date on which symptoms were first reported to GP' included on referral forms to aid consultants, give an overview and hasten the reforms that patients deserve
- national referral protocols and standardised referral forms with tick-boxes as a short-term solution, with self-referral 'one-stop-shop' clinics for all common cancers as the ultimate goal
- rapid access to the latest investigative techniques, with accurate findings

- clinic capacities to reflect need
- to be offered test results to view as a right, not a privilege.

Consent

Before giving consent, patients should be told about the cancer, all treatment options and *all* serious short- and long-term side-effects, no matter how small the risk. Only patients themselves can fully assess the risks and implications, because only they know how these might affect the quality of their lives. We also need fail-safe measures to ensure that patients are not entered in clinical trials without consent.

- Weeping men have recounted how they were not warned about incontinence and impotence.
- A professional singer was not told that treatment could affect her voice.
- Some women are unable to have sexual intercourse, some have every kind of -ostomy, and others have lost limbs.

  None of the women on the ward knew about their right to refuse student participation. A woman in her eighties with a gynaecological cancer was regularly in tears after the consultant visited with an entourage.

In order to help to remove any doctor–patient imbalance of power and reduce complaints we need:

- consent forms to be designed by patients
- forms which allow patients to choose whether or not student doctors, or doctors continuing their education, are allowed to take an active part in their care
- the consent *process* to be witnessed independently and tape-recorded
- patients to be given copies of completed forms and tapes.

  Honesty is an ethical imperative which is fundamental to any social contract ... can we justify doctors being the one group in society exempt from this fundamental role in human relationships? Any deception infringes the autonomy of the patient – the patient's right to know.[5]

Treatment

NHS Executive guidance[6] offers chilling evidence of the lack of imaging and staging for gynaecological cancers in the UK, while admitting that these are essential for determining appropriate treatment. The consequences of over- and under-treatment affect long-term survival and morbidity, with implications for fertility and sexual relationships.

Pathology may be the backbone of health services, yet a graduate trainee bio-medical scientist's starting salary is around £14 657, rising to £19 284 when they are qualified. Critical staffing levels mean unacceptable workloads, with some microbiologists and histopathologists regularly working a 60-hour week.

Although modernisation of pathology services is able to build on Audit Commission reviews, it seems that optimum use of chemotherapy will only be made cost- and treatment-effective when investment is made in advancing diagnostic technology.[7]

In 1997, a national audit of waiting times for radiotherapy showed that '25% of UK patients wait more than the four-week "maximum waiting time" set by the Joint Council for Clinical Oncology (36% for Northern and Yorkshire)'.[8] A recent study also reflected staff and equipment shortages, and reported lung cancer patients waiting up to 107 days for treatment after diagnosis (one in five cases becoming inoperable).[9] With the Royal College of Radiologists recommending four linear accelerators per million head of population,[4] it is not sufficient merely to replace those which regularly break down.

Some surgeons will not recognise 'cording' (a shortened ligament which can result in permanently restricted arm movement) and block access to physiotherapy. Effective treatment for lymphoedema needs to be started early, but patients can wait weeks to see a lone specialist nurse.

> After breast surgery, I woke to find a cannula in my 'bad' hand. The senior nurse manager denied any risk of lymphoedema from sterile needles, even though the leaflet given to breast cancer patients mentioned this.

Treatment can be arbitrary and accepted in ignorance: 'As your breasts are so small, you might as well have a mastectomy' (*General Surgeon, 1999*).

For nine weeks a woman repeatedly asked her GP for a referral. Private tests confirmed that she had breast cancer. After 12 weeks of chemotherapy and unrelieved vomiting she had lost 3 stone in weight. The oncology nurse often took days to answer her distress calls, and her suspicions of liver involvement were ignored. Private tests once more proved positive. She discovered hospitals having some success in treating liver cancers, but the oncology nurse told her 'You can take yourself all round the country – you won't get any better treatment than here.' Weeks later she was to be put on a different chemotherapy regimen, but feared that she would not survive it. 'They stood at the foot of the bed arguing. The general surgeon suggested certain drugs, but the oncology nurse said, "You can't give that intravenously!" He seemed to be learning on me.' Later still she had laparoscopic oophorectomy, and took six hours to come round from the anaesthetic. Eventually she saw an oncologist who admitted her and performed CT scans, but she died within days, leaving behind two little girls.

We need:

- pathologists and other doctors to be valued, supported and adequately resourced
- minimal delay between initial investigation and treatment
- access to specialist surgeons and oncologists
- appropriate pretreatment imaging/staging
- the management of cancers to comply with national disease-specific clinical protocols
- state-of-the-art treatment technology
- *genuine* multidisciplinary teams based on equity, whose members all meet regularly *and are willing to 'share' their patients*
- a contact nurse for outpatients as well as inpatients
- greater staff and patient awareness of potential postoperative complications
- adequate self-referral clinics for postoperative complications.

Pain relief and palliative care

People have been denied pain relief even when they pleaded for it, but cancer patients usually feel too vulnerable to complain. They may think that they are expected to put up with pain, or suffer in silence if they feel that information is limited to their assessed coping capabilities.[3] Patients should be enabled to talk about pain frequently, as needs change, so that they do not feel ashamed about asking for help. A clinical trial parallel quality-of-life study showed that 'clinicians undoubtedly under-reported morbidity'.[10]

- A lung drain was left in place for an extra 24 hours because there was 'no doctor available ... due to clinical audit', and adhered tissue was pulled out when it was removed.
- The screams of a woman whose breast was clamped to a machine for a biopsy and of a man with a closed urethra who was forcibly catheterised were ignored.

I asked for analgesia before fine-needle aspiration of a breast lump, but was told I would 'just have to put up with it'. The needle moved around over 20 times.

Fine-needle aspiration is 'a way of getting a sample of cells from a lump, usually done under local anaesthetic'.[11] (*Patient information glossary*)

Immediately following 4 weeks' aggressive treatment, a rectal examination was carried out by force (in an anal cancer patient), although the protocol allowed an 8-week healing break.

> If examination were necessary *at that time*, the only recourse would be general anaesthetic. (*Independent oncologists*)

We need:

- effective symptom control
- analgesia or anaesthetic offered for painful procedures
- adequate pain relief (from the patient's perspective)
- equally high standards of specialist palliative care in hospitals, hospices and the community.

Allied humanitarian issues

- A terminally ill patient with bowel cancer, whose 88-year-old husband was deaf, was terrified of being unable to access night-time help.
- Forty per cent of departments surveyed expect patients to walk partly naked across planning and treatment rooms, and allow open access into the room during planning sessions.[12]
- I had diarrhoea for months. Usually there was no toilet paper. (*Outpatient*)
- The wall partitioning male and female toilets stopped at the shared window recess. Men often left their door open as they urinated. Both sexes shared the single wash-basin, and the outer door had no lock. (*Inpatient*)
- I could not swallow. Nobody told me about artificial saliva ... I had terrible headaches but had to look after my screaming two-year-old while my wife tried to earn enough to keep five of us. (*Head cancer patient*)

We need:

- routine mechanisms in all departments for advising patients about ancillary services and state benefits
- gowns and changing cubicles for radiotherapy sessions
- adequate provision of single-sex, well-maintained toilets with private washing facilities
- adequate community nursing and sitter services.

Communication and information

Communication problems are widespread.[13] Improved communication between lead clinicians, including GPs, is essential to ensure that care can be consistent, side-effects anticipated and conflicting advice avoided. Most cancer patients want more information,[14–16] but doctors are often reluctant to talk about uncomfortable issues.[17] Is this for our sake or theirs? Barriers to open communication and the difficulties of facing reality when unable to cure have been deftly described by Dr Robin Carmichael,[18] along with coping strategies:

> We remain in complete control . . . we use jargon we hope they won't properly understand; we adopt an artificially cheerful exterior, signalling 'don't ask serious questions'; we use euphemisms deliberately intending to deceive (rather than to soften the blow); we lie; we pass the buck. Could it be that we are just the teeniest bit afraid of death ourselves?

To a cancer patient (with acutely charged senses), the cover-up may be less than convincing, as words, nuances, inflections, hesitations and body language are all analysed many times in the days following a consultation. The discrepancies mount up. The deceit is hurtful, demoralising and humiliating. Anything less than the truth (even lying by default) risks the destroying of trust at a time when it is desperately needed – and smiles are no substitute. Patients are still abruptly given a cancer diagnosis and sent home, or left alone on the ward, without any support or information – even when there is a cancer care centre available. Some doctors tell the relatives when an elderly (but wholly 'competent') person is terminally ill, but do not tell the patient. Sometimes information about support groups which are not hospital led is deliberately withheld.

Restricting information can:

- create acute stress
- cause frustration, resentment and depression
- block communication
- damage the doctor–patient relationship
- invite non-compliance
- result in neglect
- prevent patients from making informed treatment and lifestyle decisions.

Good communication needs to be taught. Novice riders kick a horse forward, but at advanced dressage level they communicate more subtly, to greater effect. Although doctors are initially taught to extract information and make judgements within a limited time, a non-judgemental approach and 'open' questions would allow far more meaningful dialogue. Patient involvement in education can bring a new perspective to clinicians at all levels. A recent Nuffield report[19] highlights the need for undergraduate and continuing education in communication skills, and gives sound recommendations for improving the consultation process, increasing patient participation in treatment decisions and improving the quality of such decisions. 'Advanced communication skills training will form part of continuing professional development programmes',[2] but will this component be purely optional?

For the average lay person, finding the right questions to ask can be like attempting a Master's degree in astrophysics. Clinicians who 'tailor' answers on an assumed 'need-to-know' basis may cause more stress than the cancer itself.[3,15] Feelings of powerlessness and frustration can lead to a numbing passivity which is likely to be misinterpreted as 'inability to assimilate further information'.

There are excellent guidelines for breaking bad news,[20] including a free video.[21] Not every cancer patient wants to know everything, but skilled questioning should enable people to express their initial preferences and later needs.

Specific aids and interventions can identify the desired level of involvement and facilitate shared decision making.[22,23] Extensive studies by Martin Tattersall and others have evaluated patients' communication preferences, including prompt sheets and taped consultations.[24]

Having to turn questions around and battle for answers can be exhausting:

> Seven years later they unwittingly drop a hint about late-radiation damage. 'Will I need a colostomy?', I ask. 'We don't know.' 'If someone had the same cancer and the same treatment as me, is it likely they would need a colostomy in the future?' Silence. They look at the floor. I summon my remaining ounce of strength and plead, '*Please. I need to know!*'. Pause ... 'Well, we always say ... better to have loved and lost ... (Stop prevaricating! What right have you to withhold information about *my* body?) ... 70–75% of people will need a colostomy at some point, yes.' At last! I am grateful, but feel cheated – it is devastating to be left wishing in retrospect, 'If only I had known, what changes would I have made?'.

Clinicians who become patients themselves may readily appreciate the need to understand the psychology of illness:

> I was unprepared for the emotional roller-coaster ride precipitated by my discussions with the hospital staff after the diagnosis. I soon realised the number of bitter pills I had unwittingly delivered to patients during my 15 years of practice.[25]

We need:

1 suspicions to be shared in order to alleviate the shock of diagnosis
2 patient-held information files with blank tapes (or a slot for one) for recording consultations, which could help patients to:
  - be sure of what was said
  - come to terms with the situation at their own pace, countering heuristics

- formulate questions in advance, thus saving consultation time
- provide a useful record for consultants.

'Good communication with our dying patients elevates our role as scientists to that of good neighbours – a worthy aim?'[18] Limiting information in the name of 'clinical judgement' is unwittingly being 'kind' to be 'cruel', and must surely risk the scorn of enlightened peers, for in today's changing culture of healthcare there is no place for thinly veiled paternalism.

Support

Cancer nurses have the potential to be invaluable sources of support, but if insufficiently trained can precipitate psychological morbidity.

> Cancer had returned for the second time. I was desolate and asked for counselling. The chemotherapy 'counsellor' sat above me on the bed, swinging her legs, and all she said was, 'Come on, Pat, you've got to be positive.'[26]

Cancer care centres can provide a high level of integrated support and ease the route to psychologists and ancillary services, but only if people are aware of them. The dedicated space should be freely accessible, not used for clinics.
We need:

1   Cancer care centre facilities available to patients, carers and staff, which include:

   - a library of leaflets, books, videos and relaxation tapes
   - interactive screens
   - Internet access and training
   - Social Security benefits advice
   - counselling
   - support group meetings
   - complementary therapies
   - group relaxation
   - therapeutic workshops (art, music, aromatherapy etc.)
   - listening skills training (for clinicians, and so that families can help each other)
   - Internet sites that are 'kite-marked' for reliability
   - complementary therapists who are suitably qualified, including any medical staff
   - flexi-space to allow optimum use, including support group meetings

2 routine mechanisms in every department for giving all cancer patients unbiased information about local and national support and sources of information
3 all cancer clinicians to update their listening skills regularly
4 counsellors and specialist nurse 'counsellors' to hold the British Association of Counsellors (BAC) Diploma or its equivalent, with 'supervision' according to BAC guidelines (i.e. not to 'offload', but to ensure monitoring of standards)
5 empathy, not sympathy
6 support, not pity.

Accommodation and environment

Admission to a cancer ward can mean being surrounded by terrifying evidence of disease progression and death ('How long before I deteriorate to that stage?'). The acknowledgement that the environment can influence the well-being of staff and patients has prompted an 'art in healthcare' movement. Chelsea and Westminster Hospital is a flagship in this area, but much can be achieved on a limited budget with a combination of imagination and commitment (e.g. Gloucester General Hospital, York District Hospital).

We need:

- accommodation where patients less often have to cope with the sights and sounds of others' suffering, as well as their own
- single-sex wards arranged for maximum privacy
- plenty of single rooms with en-suite facilities
- patient involvement in every aspect of planning and service delivery.

Transport

The side-effects of treatment can include sickness, diarrhoea and pain. Patients have suffered extended journeys in inappropriate transport. Despite recent improvements, 'there is no room for complacency',[27] and site specialisation will have an impact on transport needs.

We need:

- a dedicated service for cancer patients
- use of cars unless this is inappropriate
- space for carers if it is required
- direct transport from home to an integrated hospital service in a single location
- rationalised booking and appointment systems.

'Postcode prescribing', ageism and other inequalities

How does it feel to be a patient who knows that a drug which could lengthen your life is not available in your area? How does it feel to be an oncologist who is no longer able to prescribe such a drug? Although the National Institute for Clinical Excellence can recommend Taxol and Taxotere and other costly chemotherapy treatments, high costs may deter primary care trusts from funding these drugs.[28]

- Chemotherapy outpatients, unlike inpatients, do not qualify for free wigs.
- Women who are taking tamoxifen as long-term medication are, unlike diabetics, not exempt from prescription charges.
- Private patients receiving chemotherapy have been given expensive and effective anti-emetic drugs, while NHS patients alongside were given only cheaper and ineffective alternatives.
- Research findings indicate that not only premenopausal but most postmenopausal breast cancer patients would benefit from chemotherapy,[29] but are they getting it?
- 'I hope you realise just how much you are costing the NHS.' (*Chemotherapy nurse to two elderly cancer patients, 2000*).

We need:

- an end to the shameful practice of arbitrarily adding 'DNR' or '555' to patients' notes
- an end to the exclusion of elderly people from screening programmes, randomised trials or treatment without sound clinical reasons. The 'cancer stigma' is exclusion enough.

We are people and we deserve kindness, compassion and respect. We need to be valued. Perhaps our greatest challenge will be to change attitudes.

The role of patient organisations in promoting change and monitoring performance

In 1996, the NHS Executive's Patient Partnership Strategy acknowledged the consumer role and, by prioritising user involvement as key to the new NHS, the Department of Health raised the profile of patient organisations.

Feedback from patient organisations can reflect waiting times, quality standards and clinical practice, and can be used to monitor local performance against national standards. Patients are involved in setting priorities and reviewing research. They contribute to clinical audit and clinical governance as part of the National Performance Framework. Resistance to such involvement can be overcome by education and training.[30]

It is widely accepted that patients must be involved from the outset of initiatives if the latter are to have credibility in the eyes of consumers. It has been stated that 'Any professional organisation producing guidance for the public without involving the public will be pilloried'[31] yet a recent patient information booklet by a breast care nurses' group had no user input and lacked details of local support groups. Although patient group pressure can result in improved service provision, such as breast clinic one-stop shops and cancer care centres, any changes are still fragmentary.

Increasingly, however, patients and doctors are discovering the mutual benefits of working together, for both can suffer as a result of the inadequacies of a system. Partnership with patients should be seen as an enabling process that is essential to gold standards of care, not as a threat to authority. Most of the Royal Colleges now have patient liaison groups (PLGs), often consisting of equal numbers of doctors and informed lay people, which discuss sensitive issues and share perspectives. This is not mere tokenism. Lay members' views are incorporated into College responses to consultation papers, and in a ground-breaking move, two lay members from the Royal College of Pathologists PLG were invited on to the Working Group producing new guidelines for post-mortem examination.[32] Not only were many of their comments and suggestions included in the final document, but also they formulated the 'consent' form and wrote the relatives' information leaflet.

Such excellent examples of collaboration could be emulated to advantage throughout cancer care and, since user involvement is key to the development of patient-centred services, it is likely that they will be. Users and health professionals already work together within the National Cancer Alliance. Now the national charity Cancerlink's CancerVOICES Project offers training not only to cancer patients and carers who want to be user representatives, but also to health professionals who want to work with them.[2] Some regional cancer co-ordinators are already inviting patient representatives to be part of quality assurance peer review teams and cancer networks.[33]

Effective user involvement will necessitate the following:

- including users at every level
- eliciting users' views by various means
- ensuring equity
- addressing issues
- providing timely feedback to participants

- using patients and carers as educators across all disciplines, at every level
- resourcing needs (information, training, networking, support)
- reimbursing travel, carer and out-of-pocket expenses.

The gap between 'them' and 'us' is narrowing as we are learning to trust each other.

References

1   Department of Health (2000) *The NHS Plan*. Department of Health, London.

2   Department of Health (2000) *The NHS Cancer Plan*. Department of Health, London.

3   Blennerhassett M (1998) Deadly charades. *BMJ*. **316**: 1890–1.

4   Spellman P, Smith I, Bruce E *et al*. (1999) *The Cancer Journey to Secondary Care of Patients with Suspected Cancer of the Colon or Lung*. Nuffield Portfolio Programme Report No 1. NHS Executive, Northern and Yorkshire R&D, The Nuffield Institute for Health and University of Leeds, Leeds.

5   Phillips M and Dawson J (1985) *Doctors' Dilemmas: medical ethics and contemporary science*. Brighton Harvester, Brighton.

6   NHS Executive (1999) *Guidance on Commissioning Cancer Services. Improving outcomes in gynaecological cancers (the manual)*. Department of Health, London.

7   Connolly C (2000) Test match. *Health Serv J*. **5706**: 24–5.

8   Faculty of Clinical Oncology (1998) *A National Audit of Waiting Times for Radiotherapy*. Royal College of Radiologists, London.

9   O'Rourke N and Edwards R (2000) Lung cancer treatment waiting times and tumour growth. *J Clin Oncol*. **12**: 141–4.

10 United Kingdom Coordinating Committee for Cancer Research (UKCCCR) (1996) Results of the UKCCCR Phase III Anal Cancer Trial; The Parallel Quality of Life Study. *UKCCCR Anal Cancer Trial Newsletter*. **February**: 4.

11 North Yorkshire Health Authority (1999) *Personal Health File*. North Yorkshire Health Authority, York.

12 Clinical Oncology Patients' Liaison Group (1999) *Making Your Radiotherapy Service More Patient-Friendly*.The Royal College of Radiologists, London.

13 Audit Commission (1993) *What Seems to be the Matter? Communication between hospitals and patients*. HMSO, London.

14 National Cancer Alliance (1996) *Patient-Centred Cancer Services? What patients say*. National Cancer Alliance, Oxford.

15 Blennerhassett M (1996) The pain of the gentle touch. *Health Serv J*. **5497**: 25.

16   Meredith C, Symonds P, Webster L *et al.* (1996) Information needs of cancer patients in West Scotland: cross-sectional survey of patients' views. *BMJ.* **313**: 724–6.

17   Fallowfield F, Ford S and Lewis S (1995) No news is not good news: information preferences of patients with cancer. *Psycho-Oncology.* **4**: 197–202.

18   Carmichael R (1993) Help! I'm dying. *Oncol. Newsletter. J York Region Cancer Org.* **12**: 13,14.

19   Georgiou A and Robinson M (1999) *What is the Scope for Improving Health Outcomes by Promoting Patient Involvement in Decision Making? A briefing and recommendations for the NHS.* Nuffield Portfolio Programme Report No 4. NHS Executive, Northern and Yorkshire R&D, The Nuffield Institute for Health and University of Leeds, Leeds.

20   Lincoln and Louth NHS Trust (1996) *Breaking Bad News: guidelines for best practice (the stages towards excellence).* Lincoln and Louth NHS Trust, Lincoln.

21   Owen OG (2000) Communicating with professionals – medical perspectives. *Cancerlink News.* **1**: 6.

22   Degner LF and Sloan JA (1992) Decision making during serious illness: what role do patients really want to play? *J Clin Epidemiol.* **45**: 941–50.

23   O'Connor AM, Rostom A, Fiset V *et al.* (1999) Decision aids for patients facing health treatment or screening decisions: systematic review. *BMJ.* **319**: 731–4.

24   Ellis PM and Tattersall MHN (1999) How should doctors communicate the diagnosis of cancer to patients? *Ann. Med.* **31**: 336–41.

25   Poulson J (1998) Bitter pills to swallow. *NEJM.* **338**: 1844.

26   Harvey P (1999) *The perils and pitfalls of positive thinking.* Paper presented at the National Conference of Cancer Self-Help Groups, Manchester, 19 June 1999.

27   Multi-Agency Working Group (1999) *Transport Services for Cancer Patients in North Yorkshire.* North Yorkshire Health Authority, York.

28   Anon. (2000) What the papers say. *Prim Care Rep.* **2**: 5–47.

29   Early Breast Cancer Trialists' Collaborative Group (1998) Polychemotherapy for early breast cancer: an overview of the randomised trials. *Lancet.* **352**: 930–42.

30   Kohner N and Leftwich A (1998) *Partnerships: a training pack for training with patients and clients.* College of Health and Health Development Partnerships, London.

31   Williams H (2000) Patients and pathologists. *ACP News.* **Summer**: 30–2.

32   Royal College of Pathologists (2000) *Guidelines for the Retention of Tissues and Organs at Post-Mortem Examination.* Royal College of Pathologists, London.

33   Cancerlink (2001) *CancerVOICES. Issue 3.* Cancerlink, London.

CHAPTER 11

Nursing and cancer care

May Bullen

Introduction

Nurses and allied health professionals deliver a large proportion of direct care to people with cancer, their families and carers. They have a significant contribution to make in improving cancer services by ensuring a coherent service through working with one another and their medical colleagues across professional and organisational boundaries. They are crucial to the delivery of a comprehensive service and central to improvements in equity and access, as well as to the supportive care that is essential to improve the quality of experience of those who are affected by cancer.

The single factor that can confound us in improving cancer care for patients, their families and carers is getting the right workforce. This means having the right people in the right place at the right time doing the right things.

This chapter will consider the implications of the cancer plan for nursing and allied health professionals in relation to the scope and capacity of the workforce to meet the Government agenda.

The NHS Cancer Plan[1] sets out to improve care by reducing risk, promoting earlier detection, faster access to treatment and equity of treatment and care, improving community services and improving the experience of people who are living with cancer. All of this has numerous implications for nursing and allied health professions, not least with regard to the organisation, management and quality of care and services, workforce planning, education, training and continuing professional development, recruitment, retention and career pathways, and leadership. The publication of national strategic nursing and allied health professions documents[2-4] provides some direction for addressing these issues. Two themes emerge from all of these documents, namely partnership and leadership.

Partnerships

It is through interdisciplinary planning and delivery of services that the greatest impact can be made on cancer. The development of cancer networks and multi-disciplinary team-working are key to this. Nursing and allied health professions must think and develop across boundaries, and this applies not just within the NHS and healthcare providers, but also to voluntary agencies, social services, professional groups and organisations and, of course, user's and carer's groups. The cancer services collaborative brings together all care providers along the patient's cancer pathway to explore the following issues:

- co-ordination of the patient journey
- improving the patient/carer experience
- optimising care delivery
- matching capacity and demand.

Nurses and allied health professionals provide a large amount of the care that is delivered along the pathway, and they are critical to achieving the above aims through working collaboratively with colleagues in challenging traditional patterns of work and testing new ideas.

Leadership

Professional leadership is essential for the organisation and delivery of care and services, for workforce planning, for education, training and continuing professional development, and for recruitment, retention and career pathways.

Bearing these two key themes of partnership and leadership in mind, what is the impact of the NHS Cancer Plan on the scope and capacity of nursing and related professions in cancer care?

Reducing risk

Health promotion and cancer prevention are the remit of all nurses and allied health professionals, and should be an integral part of all care. However, this will require a change of mind set and the application of wider thinking within cancer services. Caring for cancer patients requires consideration of the entire family unit. A diagnosis of cancer in the family often prompts other family members to consider their own lifestyles. Specific examples of this include smoking and diet.

Smoking

All health professionals have responsibility for contributing to smoking reduction initiatives in partnership with one another. Although most smoking reduction initiatives are the domain of community staff, health professionals working within cancer services should be aware of local initiatives so that they can direct people towards them.

Diet

Nurses in particular are at the forefront of dietary advice and guidance. Changing diet for one member of a family often results in dietary changes for all the other members. Nurses must work in partnership with dietitians not only in relation to dietary assessment but also in finding opportunities for family health promotion. Low fruit and vegetable intake within a family can be due to a number of reasons, including socio-economic factors. A well-informed, wider-thinking nurse may be crucial to enabling lifestyle changes that will alter attitudes and thus protect future generations.

Raising awareness

Nurses and allied health professionals have major opportunities to raise the public's awareness of the contribution of diet and healthy lifestyle to reducing the risk of cancer, as well as their knowledge of the symptoms of cancer. As cancer affects one in three members of the population, non-cancer nurses and allied health professionals are in an excellent position to identify individuals with symptoms suggestive of cancer. A nurse or allied health professional may be the first professional to identify someone with a high suspicion of cancer. Although primary care is considered to play the major role here, it may be a nurse or allied health professional in secondary, tertiary or palliative care to whom a relative first talks about a problem. The public expects health professionals to have knowledge both of the symptoms and of the process for referral into appropriate services. However, this has training implications.

Earlier detection

The cancer plan identifies two main areas for improvement, namely improved screening and referral guidance.

People who enter screening programmes are aware that the reason for the screening is to detect cancer, and therefore anxiety levels are raised in these individuals. With the extension of screening programmes there will be an increase in the number of people who require support and information. As new screening pilots and extended programmes develop, experience from breast and cervical screening needs to be taken into account. These programmes demonstrate that there are also issues related to management of the anxieties of individuals who are not included in screening programmes and pilots. Professional leadership is necessary to ensure that appropriate support is available for all.

Faster access to treatment

Rapid access from primary to secondary care for breast cancer has placed a strain on resources. This is partly due to public expectations, as patients know that a lump in the breast could be cancer and that a person with the possibility of cancer should be seen by a specialist within two weeks. This has now been extended to other cancers.

Partnership between professionals and services, as well as professional leadership, are necessary in order to ensure that services develop safely with adequately prepared staff.

With the need to get people through the system more quickly, the opportunity arises for nurses and allied health professionals to play a larger part in diagnosis. This may be by taking a role in assessment and ordering of investigations, thereby freeing doctors' time for interpreting results and making diagnoses. This can be achieved by the setting up of nurse-run clinics where nurses are clerking patients and undertaking investigations that were previously undertaken by doctors (e.g. endoscopy, biopsy, aspirations). Diagnostic radiographers are already beginning to undertake some procedures (e.g. barium enemas) and are reporting findings. The training implications for these developments involve medical practitioners as well as nurses and other clinical professionals, and have the potential to increase waiting times initially, as the practice element of training is time-consuming for all concerned. It takes longer to coach someone in a procedure than for experienced practitioners to undertake it themselves.

In developing new roles, particularly for nurses, it is important that this is not achieved at the expense of nursing. There is potential here for nursing roles to become technician roles and for the core elements of nursing to be lost. Strong leadership is required to ensure that this does not happen. There need to be clear job descriptions, flexible jobs and robust protocols to ensure accountability and safe practice.

Reducing waiting times has the potential to reduce anxiety, but it also has the potential to reduce patients' feelings of control and involvement. It is vital to ensure that patients have the support and information necessary to make informed choices about their treatment when time spans are reduced. This has resource implications, as making an informed choice at a time of crisis and stress (a diagnosis of cancer) frequently requires time and skilled support. A single interview that is filled with verbal and written information is not enough. Specialist nurses/radiographers who undertake this frequently report that they are over-stretched. Service delivery and resources need to be scrutinised carefully.

Equity of treatment and care

The national cancer standards[5] that have been developed are mainly about the structure of cancer services, and will be used as a basis for the accreditation or appraisal of services. However, regions are keen to take the opportunity to make the exercise of peer review more than just a 'tick-box' exercise. Accreditation visits lead to agreed plans for development, and resources will be allocated to meet the plans. It is therefore vital that nurses and allied health professionals on the ground (i.e. those who are with the patients and their families and really know how the disease and service provision is affecting them) contribute to the process. A large part of the standards concentrates on multidisciplinary teamworking. Specialist nurses have a key co-ordinating role in the multidisciplinary team, ensuring that patients have appropriate support and that they also provide continuity of care as patients move between services. The specialist nurse makes a valuable contribution to decision making about treatment and care. The relationship that is developed between a patient and the nurse enables the patient to make informed choices about their treatment and care, and also enables the nurse to contribute relevant psychosocial information to the clinical team. Effective teams are about effective partnerships – not only between disciplines but also between services, and the specialist nurse has a pivotal role in this.

The development of clinical outcomes guidance on specific cancers[6] and the National Institute for Clinical Excellence guidance on cancer treatments will continue to have implications for workforce planning related to treatment delivery and patient support through treatment. Emerging guidance needs to be viewed with this in mind.

Nurses and allied health professionals must seek opportunities to contribute to the cancer research portfolio. Competing for funding is not easy, and medicine has a lot more support behind it from pharmaceutical companies than do other health professionals. However, the quality of the patient experience is high on the new agenda, and this provides new opportunities. There are a number of areas other than treatment outcomes that need to be researched (e.g. the effect of multidisciplinary team care on patient outcomes, and the effect of a changed organisation of care on patient and family outcomes).

Improving community services

Cancer patients spend most of their lives at home. The start of the cancer pathway is in primary care, and patients then dip in and out of secondary and tertiary care as they travel the path. Yet primary care has tended to view its role in cancer care mainly in terms of the palliative stage. There are opportunities for far greater involvement in shared care as patients undergo treatment. Early discharge post surgery is well accepted as a way of better utilising precious surgical beds. This has major resource implications for both surgical postoperative care and information and support to help patients to make informed choices about their future treatment and care. Chemotherapy may be another area for shared care development in order to reduce attendance at chemotherapy units and thereby increase chemotherapy delivery capacity.

Primary care also has an important future in follow-up. Much of this could be nurse led, but clear protocols detailing responsibility and accountability will be required.

The availability of co-ordinated 24-hour community services for patients with advanced cancer is a challenge and requires clear definition in order to avoid abuse. Marie-Curie nurses have undertaken specific cancer care training and provide invaluable care for patients in their own homes, enabling them to stay at home rather than being admitted to hospital or a hospice. Community Macmillan nurses and hospice community specialist palliative care nurses also provide support and symptom management for patients in their own homes. Community and practice nurses, as part of the primary healthcare team, provide non-specialist care and support for cancer patients and their families. It is essential that all care providers work in partnership to improve services in the community, maximise existing resources and ensure that services meet individuals' needs. This requires co-ordination, which is a role for nursing.

Improving the experience of patients living with cancer

National strategic direction for supportive care falls into three main areas:

- information
- psychosocial support
- specialist palliative care.

This is the domain not just of hospices and specialist palliative care providers, but of all professionals who care for patients with cancer and their families.

There is a need to look at the available NHS, voluntary and social services across cancer networks and the skills within them, and to determine how the collective resources can be used most efficiently to ensure that patients' needs are met.

There is also a need to assess and record effectively the supportive care needs of *all* cancer patients. Currently this is a hit-and-miss affair depending on service configuration. It is probably best in breast services for patients who enter service through dedicated breast clinics with breast care nurse involvement, but is not so effective for patients who enter the service via other routes. Patients who are referred to palliative care services also have a better chance of having their supportive care needs assessed, but they may have travelled a long way along a pathway before palliative care becomes part of their care.

Assessing and meeting supportive care needs are a new challenge. Nursing can lead this development, investing in partnerships with NHS healthcare providers, voluntary agencies, social services, professional groups and organisations, and users and carers. Macmillan nurses and other cancer clinical nurse specialists are in a key position to undertake this, as they have the knowledge and skills necessary to assess holistic needs and refer or direct patients to appropriate services.

Organisation of care

Networks are mentioned a number of times in the Cancer Plan. These are best described as virtual organisations that manage cancer care (i.e. managed clinical networks). They consist of providers who provide care for cancer patients and also commissioners of that care. Initially, providers of cancer care were considered to be cancer units and cancer centres, and commissioners were health authorities. However, since the emergence of primary care trusts there is a new challenge of how to integrate them into the network. A large amount of cancer care in the community is and will be provided by nurses. Professional leadership here is essential to ensure that the development of services in both the community and acute sectors does not occur at the expense of elements of care. All networks should have a lead nurse as well as a lead clinician and lead manager. The role of the network lead team is strategic leadership, with responsibility for the development and implementation of the network service delivery plan. The network lead nurse has specific areas of responsibility, which include the following:

- integrating general, site-specific and palliative care nursing which is based on research, knowledge and experience

- establishing working links with specialist nurses from the network disease site-specific groups
- assessing workforce demands, training and support needs, and developing common education strategies with local Workforce Confederations and education providers
- ensuring network working relationships and communication with nurses and allied health professionals in primary, secondary and tertiary areas and hospices
- ensuring that network-wide user perspective informs the development of cancer services
- encouraging teaching and research in cancer and palliative care across the network.

With this large remit it is essential that network lead nurses have sufficient dedicated time, as well as the skills necessary to lead the care agenda across the network within a changing culture of decision making.

Workforce development

Existing services must be designed and planned to take account of future staffing demands, skill mix requirements and education and development needs.

Although the Cancer Plan offers 20 000 additional nurses and 6500 additional allied health professionals, these will not appear overnight. Emerging new roles and skill mixes challenge traditional roles. Not only are nurses and allied health professionals undertaking traditionally medical roles, but also nursing and allied health professional helper roles are emerging.

These developments offer a challenge to education and development. Nurses and allied health professionals need to have knowledge and skills appropriate to their area of care along the pathway. New courses may need to be developed, and existing courses may need to be delivered in different ways. Taking the workforce away from the workplace is not compatible with providing a service. Education and training need to be provided in the workplace through practice. There is a great deal of in-house training that takes place. The challenge is to harness this to overall education and training through partnerships between service and education providers, and to ensure consistent outcomes. The framework for nursing educational preparation identified in *Making a Difference*[3] has been applied to cancer nursing in *The Nursing Contribution to Cancer Care*.[4] Pre-registration education needs to strengthen the cancer component so that all nurses have a better understanding of the needs of cancer patients and their families. Registered nurses who have not undertaken specialist education should seek advice and refer to specialist nurses. Registered nurses who are working within the speciality are expected to undertake further specialist education to degree level in order to become cancer nurses. Senior registered cancer nurses are expected to be pursuing a pathway to Masters degree level, and consultant nurses should hold at least a Masters degree. This framework is applicable to allied health professionals, and the development of multidisciplinary programmes will enable senior registered cancer practitioners and consultant practitioners to emerge in all disciplines.

It is vital that nurses and allied health professionals are supported by their own profession as we move into this brave new world. They need to be actively involved in recruitment and retention strategies for the workforce that cares for cancer patients, wherever they are along the pathway.

The Nursing Contribution to Cancer Care states that 'The role and contribution of nursing to cancer care is vital at every level and at every stage of the cancer journey for those affected by cancer.' This is also true for the allied health professions.

Through partnership and leadership, nursing and allied health professions can and must influence the experience of those who are affected by cancer.

References

1 Department of Health (2000) *The NHS Cancer Plan: a plan for investment, a plan for reform.* Department of Health, London.

2 Department of Health (2000) *Meeting the Challenge: a strategy for the allied health professionals.* Department of Health, London.

3 Department of Health (1999) *Making a Difference: strengthening the nursing, midwifery and health visiting contribution to health and healthcare.* Department of Health, London.

4 Department of Health (2000) *The Nursing Contribution to Cancer Care: a strategic programme of action in support of the national cancer programme.* Department of Health, London.

5 Department of Health (2000) *Manual of Cancer Services Standards.* Department of Health, London.

6 Department of Health (1996–2000) *Guidance on Commissioning Cancer Services. Improving Outcomes in Cancer series.* Department of Health, London.

CHAPTER 12

Palliative care

Anne Garry

Introduction

The specialist elements of palliative care, the hospice movement and pain control are not unique to cancer, but they do play a major role in determining the quality of care and patient expectations in the end-stage of the disease. Palliative care has a broader remit than 'care for the dying'. Good palliative care should be an integral part of the care of every patient, irrespective of the stage of their illness, and may contribute towards improving the health of the population. It should interface in a seamless way with all cancer treatment services and primary care to provide the best quality of life for the patient and their family.[1,2] It differs in philosophy from curative strategies in that it focuses primarily on the consequences of a disease rather than its cause or specific cure. It recognises that important work takes place around patients, their families and front-line health care professionals. This is essential to cancer care. It has recently been put on to the political agenda through the NHS Cancer Plan[3] and the strategic framework for palliative care[4] is eagerly awaited.

> It is the right of every person with a life-threatening illness to receive appropriate palliative care wherever they are and at whatever stage of their illness.[5]

Evolution of palliative care services

Hospices date from the nineteenth century (St Joseph's Hospice was established by the Irish Sisters of Charity), but the 'modern' hospice came into being in 1967 when Dame Cicely Saunders set up St Christopher's Hospice in Sydenham, London.[4] The movement has largely grown outside the NHS, and services in the past have been fragmented. Some hospices have developed in an ad hoc fashion through voluntary effort and fundraising, but the needs of

---

Box 12.1: Statement of definitions

Palliative care is the active total care of patients whose disease is not respon-sive to curative treatment. Control of pain, of other symptoms, and of psy-chological, social and spiritual problems is paramount. (World Health Organisation, 1990)

Palliative care
- affirms life and regards dying as a normal process
- neither hastens nor postpones death
- provides relief from pain and other symptoms
- integrates the psychological and spiritual aspects of patient care
- offers a support system to help patients to live as actively as possible until their death
- offers a support system to help the family to cope during the patient's illness and in their own bereavement.

A *palliative care approach* aims to promote physical, psychological, social and spiritual well-being, and is informed by a set of key palliative care principles.

Palliative care principles
- focus on quality of life, which includes good symptom control
- whole-person approach, taking into account the person's past life experience and current situation
- care which encompasses both the person with life-threatening disease and those who matter to the person
- respect for patient autonomy and choice (e.g. with regard to place of care, treatment options, access to specialist palliative care)
- emphasis on open and sensitive communication, which extends to patients, informal carers and professional colleagues.

Palliative interventions
These are non-curative treatments given by specialists in disciplines other than specialist palliative care, aimed at controlling distressing symptoms and improving the patient's quality of life (e.g. through the use of pallia-tive radiotherapy, chemotherapy, medical and surgical procedures, and anaesthetic techniques for pain relief).

Specialist palliative care
Specialist palliative care services are those with palliative care as their core speciality. They demand a high level of professional skill from trained staff, and are required by a significant minority of people whose deaths are anticipated.

the population were not necessarily taken into account, and a home care service or a day hospice may well have been more appropriate. The Calman–Hine Report[1] has acknowledged that there should be much more collaboration, partnership and communication between all providers of cancer care and palliative care. The hospice movement is responsible for developing the practice of palliative care, looking after patients with cancer and other life-threatening illnesses. In 1987, palliative medicine was formally recognised as a subspecialty by the Royal College of Physicians.

Health authorities were first asked by the Department of Health to work together with local palliative care providers in 1987, and this has since climbed up the NHS policy agenda.

In 1996, an NHS Executive letter[2] summarised the impact of the Calman–Hine Report on cancer care services. Its aim was to ensure that the benefits and advances in palliative care were available to all patients wherever they happened to be.

In 1998, a Department of Health circular[6] asked health authorities and primary care groups to draw up palliative care strategies. Two years later, only one-third of health authorities had produced one. However, palliative care principles should become integral to the whole of NHS practice and be available to all patients, irrespective of disease.

Palliative care is a key element of NHS modernisation, such as the national service frameworks on cancer,[3] coronary heart disease,[7] mental health[8] and services for older people.[9]

The NHS Plan[10] states that health services, in partnership with other agencies, need to make high-quality palliative and supportive care available to those older people who need it. Clearly this will have an impact on palliative care services, and resources would need to follow.

Current provision

The voluntary and charity sector provides most of the hospice and specialist palliative care, including around 75% of inpatient hospice units, representing 2600 beds.[11,12] The NHS manages 56 acute palliative care units, providing 6000 beds. All hospice care is provided free of charge. An estimated 56 000 admissions are made to hospices each year. Around 29 000 people die in specialist palliative care units annually, including 19% of all cancer deaths.

The number of community specialist palliative care teams has trebled in the last decade, and 135 000 people receive palliative home care every year, and around 50% of deaths occur at home when these teams are involved with patients. Around 90% of patients who receive care from a Marie-Curie nurse die at home.[13]

A total of 28 000 new patients attend specialist palliative day care services every year.

The number of palliative care teams based in hospitals has increased rapidly, reaching 275 in the UK by July 1996. The aim is to have a team in all cancer units and centres.[14]

Influences on the shaping of services

Visiting Regional Cancer Working Groups have influenced the shaping of cancer and palliative care services. Their role has been to visit cancer units and centres to ascertain that the Calman–Hine initiatives have been implemented. Some areas of practice are well developed but others need much attention. A needs assessment should be conducted and used to inform the palliative care strategy.[15] Guidance may be drawn from a number of National Council for Hospice and Specialist Palliative Care Services documents[16,17] and the awaited strategic framework. A lead clinician in palliative care should be appointed and nominated to attend regional cancer networks and local cancer steering groups, and to lead the local palliative care strategy group.

The palliative care strategy group members should include providers of specialist palliative care, strategic health authorities and primary care organisation personnel involved in the Cancer Health Improvement and Modernisation Programme (HIMP), hospital trusts, social services and the community health council or successor body. The function of the palliative care strategy group is to consult with and inform acute trusts, primary care trusts and strategic health authorities about local practice and the way in which the services should be developed. It is important that any new developments fit into the overall Palliative Care Strategy as part of the Cancer Network Service Delivery Plan, the local Cancer Health Improvement and Modernisation Programme and cancer unit's strategy to prevent duplication or fragmentation of services. The role of the group is to develop clear referral and treatment pathways, including a palliative care formulary and a cancer and palliative care directory. It is involved both in devising an education strategy district-wide for palliative care, and in information and communication issues.

Current costings

It is estimated that current services cost around £300 million per year, and that the voluntary sector provides up to 60% of this from charitable resources as well as most of the capital stock of premises and equipment, which runs into millions of pounds. It is estimated that a further £150 million will be required as a minimum investment to implement some of the basic services.[3,15] Arrangements between NHS commissioners and the voluntary sector of hospice and specialist palliative care will need to be developed to look at funding issues. Any new resources should only be directed at palliative care services which are based on need and have been planned collaboratively with NHS trusts, primary care trusts, social services and the palliative care providers.

Funding

Acute hospital trusts, community trusts and hospices are providers of specialist palliative care. The ultimate aim is to promote partnership and collaboration, and future developments should be discussed with primary care trusts, the acute hospitals' trust and providers of specialist palliative care. The possible options for joint initiatives should be explored by approaching charitable organisations such as Cancer Relief, Macmillan, local cancer charities, independent hospices and lottery application boards, and applying for government monies targeted at cancer services. Health authorities with a socially deprived area and significant ethnic minority were eligible to apply for the Government's new opportunities fund (NOF), 'Living with Cancer'.[18]

Supportive care strategy

Each district should have a specialist resource for both primary care and hospital-based services. This facility should work with local hospital and oncology services and with the primary care teams to allow good communication and rapid access to specialised palliative treatments for symptom control, to provide respite care and to give psycho-oncology support to the patient and their family at all stages, including bereavement. The role of primary care services in the delivery of high-quality care to patients is vital. Specialist services in both hospital and the community are to empower the skills of the primary health care team and hospital teams, and not to deskill them!

Box 12.2: Role of palliative care in the primary-care-led NHS

- symptom control for all patients (holistic care)
- empowering professionals with regard to the management of dying

- recognising and supporting the skills of GPs
- providing alternatives to fast-paced and sometimes thoughtlessly invasive acute hospital services.

Multiprofessional teams should be available in all care settings, but this has yet to be achieved. The multiprofessional palliative care teams should include trained specialist medical and nursing staff, social workers, physiotherapists and occupational therapists, and should have access to other professional services such as dietetics, speech and language therapy, chaplaincy, psychology, psychiatry, pain team and a lymphoedema specialist. Patient and relative facilities should ensure privacy and dignity, with rooms for confidential discussions, and allow relatives to remain with very ill patients. Spiritual care should also be available when required.[19] This should result in a smooth progression of care between home, hospital and hospice (*see* Figure 12.1).

Palliative care in the context of the National Cancer Strategy will hopefully be a priority within the developing Supportive Care Strategy, but it needs to be cast wider than that in order to reflect the aims of HSC 1998/115,[6] namely for all healthcare professionals, NHS commissioners of healthcare and the Department of Health to respond to 'the right of every person with a life-threatening illness to receive appropriate palliative care'.

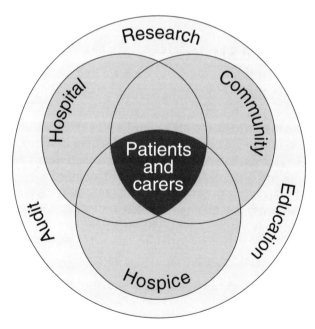

Figure 12.1:   Model of palliative care.

- To ensure that access to specialist services is available in all care settings, there should be sufficient numbers of appropriately trained specialists in palliative care.
- All healthcare workers should practise the palliative care approach as well as providing support at all stages of cancer.
- Support and advice from specialist services should be available 24 hours a day. Access for patients with cancer should be equitable.
- Access to specialist services for patients with non-cancer diagnoses should be provided according to need on a basis that is comparable to that for patients with cancer.
- A core service should be available to any given population.

The challenges

The challenges identified by the Government are reflected in the following priorities for palliative care, and build on the modernisation principles[10] for the NHS:

- improving patient care (both access and empowerment)
- building partnerships to provide seamless care
- performance (ensuring common standards and value for money)
- prevention and reduced inequality
- making better use of the professions.

Improving patient care

Access

Not all patients and their families have access to good and consistent palliative care throughout the patient journey. This may hinder the achievement of a 'good death'. The 1999 survey[18] revealed major regional variations in access to palliative care, and did not reflect the level of need (e.g. there were differences in the incidence of cancer deaths, in the levels of ethnic and other minorities, and in the levels of social and economic deprivation or the resources available). Regions with fewer resources appear to achieve greater access than others with greater resources. More research is needed to understand these issues.

It is essential to map through postcodes all palliative care and cancer services across catchment populations of each specialist palliative care provider in both voluntary and statutory sectors in order to collect more accurate statistics and help future planning of services. Future minimum data sets should include postcodes.

Patient empowerment

Patients and their relatives should be fully informed about diagnosis, treatment and care options and the services available for care and support, a view which is endorsed by the National Cancer Alliance.[20] This is particularly important for people from diverse ethnic and cultural backgrounds.[21] Offering the choice of care at home or in other settings is essential. Involving relatives and carers (if the patient wishes) and supporting carers are also requirements.

Patient-held records, telephone helplines, cancer information centres with easily accessible written information, videos and Internet technology are all helping patients and their carers to improve their knowledge of the illness.

Patient choice at the end of life

Recent evidence shows that patients wish to be cared for and to die in their own homes if possible.[13] However, for some an appropriate inpatient setting is preferred to a home death. Good home deaths require access to a range of specialist palliative care and primary care services, committed GPs and district nurses, and good co-ordination with social services. Access to education for health and social care professionals is essential in order to maintain high-quality home care.

Services should include the following:

- flexibility, to give the patient real choice with regard to care options and place of care and death, and to provide quality in the last days of life
- readily available information on services that are offered locally
- alternatives to hospital care
- equity of access to hospice and specialist palliative care
- bereavement support for carers and families.

Building partnership

Hospice and specialist palliative care services provide support to services for all disease and patient groups. Currently they are primarily focused on patients with a cancer diagnosis, but increasingly they offer services to those with a non-cancer diagnosis (5–24%).

In most health authority areas, the hospice and specialist palliative care services (SPCS) components are provided by a range of different agencies across the NHS, the voluntary sector and social services.

Specific advice was set out in HSC 1999/023[22] for health and social service authorities to build relationships with the voluntary sector. A palliative care service model capable of delivering high-quality services should have NHS and voluntary sector providers and commissioners working collaboratively in partnership.

Developing services through partnership

- Palliative care strategies should be based on local needs assessments.
- Acute services should assess the rate of deaths and assess the level of palliative care needed.
- The training of nursing home staff in palliative care should be improved and maintained by developing link nurse posts specifically to support and empower the residents and staff of nursing homes.
- There should be further development of Macmillan GP facilitators to enhance the palliative care provided by primary healthcare teams.
- Access to responsive services should be open to all who need them, when and where they need them.
- Information about treatment and care options should be made available so that patients and families are able to exercise personal choice over their care and where it takes place.
- The palliative care skills and knowledge of healthcare professionals in primary, secondary and tertiary care should be enhanced.
- SPCS should be available in all care settings, including nursing homes.
- A range of inpatient care should be available, including specialist and intermediate palliative care.
- Advice and support should be available 24 hours a day.

Intermediate care

Intermediate care is a whole-system approach to a range of multiprofessional, multi-agency services designed to promote independence by:

- reducing avoidable admissions to acute hospitals
- facilitating timely discharge from acute hospitals and promoting effective rehabilitation
- minimising dependence on long-term care in institutional settings
- employing clear admission and discharge criteria for the use of intermediate-care beds.

Nationally, intermediate-care bed development involves the use of community hospital and nursing home beds. These are essentially generic beds and will need to be supported by additional educational input and nursing, and may require specialist palliative care input.

Performance and service evaluation (standards and value for money)

- Standards and performance indicators should be developed which apply to commissioners of palliative care services and to the NHS Executive, as well as to the providers of services in both the NHS and the voluntary sector.[3,16,23]
- The National Council is developing national standards, performance indicators and related minimum data sets.
- It is necessary to ensure that effective systems of performance management for the national standards are implemented across the NHS and the voluntary sector.
- Clinical governance arrangements need to be introduced into voluntary sector services which are compatible with those implemented in the NHS.

Role of palliative care networks

This includes the following:

- development of eligibility criteria for patients who require specialist palliative care
- monitoring the quality of palliative care services
- ensuring that the health authorities develop palliative care strategies for inclusion in the local Health Improvement Programmes
- ensure equity of:
  - access to SPCS across the network
  - workforce skills in palliative care across the network
- training and research development to include educational programmes for health and social care providers and patients about the availability and benefits of palliative care services.

Box 12.3:   Performance aims in palliative care

1   *Fair access and timeliness*. All patients with palliative care needs have access to palliative care services when they need them.
2   *Effectiveness*. All patients have their symptoms managed to a degree that is acceptable to them, and achievable by multiprofessional team intervention within the limits of current palliative care knowledge.
3   *Patient/carer experience*. The patient and their family/carers are provided with the information that they require relating to diagnosis and

progress of disease, care options and support services, thus enabling them to make informed choices. The family members/carers receive psychological, emotional, spiritual, social or practical support which is responsive to their perception of their needs.

4 *Communication between professionals.* There is effective communication within the specialist and hospice palliative care teams and with other agencies, providing continuity of care and support for patients, their families and carers.

5 *Efficiency.* The resources that are employed to produce the desired outcomes for patients and their families are the minimum required in order to achieve that.

6 *Health outcome.*

Prevention through palliative care

Health outcome

Improvement in health at the end of life is as important and worthwhile as that at any other stage of life. It is also relevant to palliative care, despite the fact that these patients invariably die, in most cases quite quickly.[32] Good palliative care may make a contribution to improvement of the health of the population by reducing the suffering of patients, maximising the quality of life of patients through good symptom control and rehabilitation, and sustaining the family and its psychological health during the patient's illness and after the death of the patient.[24] Palliative and supportive care is a core priority in health and social care services.

'How a patient dies lives on in the memory of their family'. This is a haunting but very powerful statement. The dead do not come back to tell us whether we have got it right, but the relatives do. A good death is important for patients and their families if it can be achieved with dignity, in the location of choice and with the patient's symptoms well managed. Good palliative care at the end of life, as well as being an appropriate compassionate response in a civilised society, also makes economic sense. Supporting families during illness and bereavement reduces potential morbidity and potentially lessens future demand on the NHS and social services.

Inequality

Unmet needs

The symptoms that cancer and non-cancer patients experience during the last year of life are much the same, namely pain, nausea, vomiting and breathlessness. Around 50% of cancer patients access palliative care services, but only 7%

of those with a non-cancer diagnosis. This is a significant gap, as the total number of non-cancer patients with symptoms is twice that of cancer patients.[25]

Another potential gap concerns the needs of ethnic minority communities,[21] as the proportion of deaths in hospices and at home are lower than among white populations.

All specialist palliative care providers should recognise that they have a role in the care of patients with advanced and progressive disease of any diagnosis and from any ethnic group, and they will need appropriate training to upgrade their skills to fulfil this role. Strategies need to respond to unmet needs.

Out-of-hours care

Most patients prefer to stay at home, yet more unnecessary admissions to acute hospitals occur at night, on bank holidays and at weekends.[26] This may be due to poor handover procedures between primary healthcare teams and emergency doctors, non-availability of appropriate emergency drugs or equipment, or lack of out-of-hours district nursing cover or specialist palliative care advisory services.

The need for out-of-hours services is minimised by anticipating patient and family needs and good care planning. The current availability of out-of-hours services across the country ranges from telephone advice to professionals, to direct care. However, most areas do not have a 24-hour range of palliative care services.

Good out-of-hours care

This is characterised by the following:

1 availability of advice and support for professionals from specialist palliative care services for:

  • telephone advice to healthcare professionals providing general palliative care with access to domiciliary visits and admission to an inpatient unit if appropriate
  • clear protocols to be devised

2 availability of general palliative care support for patients and families for:

  • telephone support from on-call medical services, district nursing services and NHS Direct
  • home visiting from medical deputising services and district nursing on-call services
  • home nursing and sitting services from voluntary and statutory services

3   education/training in the palliative care approach
4   two-way handover systems to and from primary care and out-of-hours services, to ensure that up-to-date information about the patient's condition is continuously available to those involved in their care (e.g. through handover forms, access to electronic messages, patient-held records)
5   availability of emergency palliative care drugs
6   access to appropriate palliative care for residents of nursing homes
7   better training in palliative care issues for all staff of nursing homes, and development of link-nurse posts to support and empower residents and staff of nursing homes.[27]

Making better use of professionals

It is the responsibility of every healthcare professional to practise the palliative care approach, and to call in specialist care colleagues if the need arises, as an integral component of good clinical practice, whatever the illness or the stage.[28]

Education/training

Each health authority should ensure that cancer and palliative care education is a high priority and that it is part of the Cancer Health Improvement and Modernisation Programme. Workforce Confederations, health trusts, primary care trusts, universities and providers of palliative and cancer care education should work in partnership to produce a curriculum that is appropriate for the workforce. All healthcare professionals need a minimum level of understanding about cancer, including doctors, nurses, allied health professionals, healthcare assistants, porters, cleaners and administrative staff such as receptionists and secretaries. Core competencies are required for all professions that are in contact with cancer patients (including social services personnel) and those on training and career pathways. It will not be possible to deliver good models of palliative care without a range of professional expertise.

Palliative care should be a compulsory part of all health and social care professional education, and training programmes, which are accredited, should be regularly evaluated. There is a palliative care curriculum for senior house officers, GP registrars and specialist registrars.

Proposals for rectifying medical, nursing and other staff shortages should take into account the additional workforce requirements that arise from any expansion of service to achieve equity of access across diagnosis and stage of disease. Professional and workforce development within palliative care and supportive care networks needs to be enhanced to improve recruitment and retention.

Palliative care networks should provide a formal means by which professionals trained in palliative care and those with specific skills in providing psychological and social support can support their colleagues throughout the care pathway and offer a co-ordinated programme of continuing education.

Doctors' education

Junior house officers, senior house officers, specialist registrars, GPs and consultants, and all doctors of the future, need exposure to the care of patients with cancer and other life-limiting illnesses so that they gain confidence in managing those who are terminally ill.

Is a one-hour lecture every six months sufficient for junior doctors? Or half a day in a GP vocational training scheme? How can this cover what a good death entails, or the supportive care aspects, or the difficult ethical issues that are encountered? Surveys of GPs,[29] GP registrars,[30] junior doctors[31] and lead clinicians[32] reveal that very little in the way of education and training was encountered, and this situation could be vastly improved.

One of the important roles of Macmillan GP facilitators is to devise a programme that is appropriate to the needs of the GPs who work alongside the palliative care professionals.

Research

Patient care, audit and research should be inextricably intertwined.[33,34] Some units are too small to conduct research in palliative care on their own, but should be willing to participate in multicentre trials and regional work. The numbers of individuals involved in palliative care in any one locality can be small, so working together makes sense. Some regions are setting up research groups attached to universities.

Achievement of the NHS Plan

It is clear that whatever shape the National Plan for Palliative Care takes, there must be robust organisational arrangements in place at a local level for implementing its recommendations.

Conclusions

These are my personal reflections, and I would like to thank all of my mentors, friends and colleagues along the way who have helped to shape the way in which I view palliative care and the way it fits into the new NHS. It is refreshing to see palliative care services developing within the hospitals and community and becoming an integrated and accepted part of medical and nursing services.

With more forward planning, collaboration and partnership, the needs of the population will be better served – hopefully in a more holistic manner. I look forward to the implementation of the NHS Cancer Plan, and am encouraged by the emphasis on the palliative and supportive care component, which until recently has not been regarded as a priority.

References

1   Department of Health (1995) *A Policy Framework for Commissioning Cancer Services: a Report by the Expert Advisory Group on Cancer to the Chief Medical Officers of England and Wales. Guidance for purchasers and providers of cancer services.* Department of Health, London.

2   NHS Executive (1996) *A Policy Framework for Commissioning Cancer Services: palliative care services.* EL (96)85. Department of Health, London.

3   Department of Health (2000) *The NHS Cancer Plan.* DoH, London.

4   National Council for Hospice and Specialist Palliative Care Services (2000) *Draft National Plan and Strategic Framework for Palliative Care, 2000–2005,* for Consultation. National Council for Hospice and Specialist Palliative Care Services, London.

5   National Council for Hospice and Specialist Palliative Care Services (1995) *Specialist Palliative Care: a statement of definitions.* Occasional Paper 8. National Council for Hospice and Specialist Palliative Care Services, London.

6   Department of Health (1998) *Palliative Care.* HSC 1998/115. Department of Health, London.

7   NHS Executive (2000) *National Service Frameworks: modern standards and service models – coronary heart disease.* HSC 2000/012. NHS Executive, Leeds.

8   Department of Health (1999) *National Framework for Mental Health: modern standards and service models for mental health.* HSC 1999/223. Department of Health, London.

9   Department of Health (2000) *National Service Framework for Older People.* The Stationary Office, London.

10 Department of Health (2000) *The NHS Plan.* The Stationery Office, London.

11 Eve A, Smith AM and Tebbit P (1997) Hospice and palliative care in the UK, 1994–5. *Palliative Med.* **11**: 31–43.

12 Clark D, Hockley J and Ahmedzai S (1997) *New Themes in Palliative Care.* Open University Press, Buckingham.

13 Wilkinson S (2000) Fulfilling patients' wishes: palliative care at home. *Int J Palliative Nurs.* 6: 212.

14 National Council for Hospice and Specialist Palliative Care Services (1996) *Palliative Care in the Hospital Setting.* Occasional Paper 10. National Council for Hospice and Specialist Palliative Care Services, London.

15 Higginson IJ (1997) Palliative and terminal care: health care needs assessment. In: A Stevens and J Raftery (eds) *The Epidemiology-Based Needs Assessment Reviews.* Second series. Radcliffe Medical Press, Oxford.

16 National Council for Hospice and Specialist Palliative Care Services (1999) *Palliative Care 2000: commissioning through partnership.* National Council for Hospice and Specialist Palliative Care Services, London.

17 National Council for Hospice and Specialist Palliative Care Services (1997) *Dilemmas and Directions: the future of specialist palliative care.* Occasional Paper 11. National Council for Hospice and Specialist Palliative Care Services, London.

18 NHS Executive (2000) *New Opportunities Fund (NOF). Living with cancer.* NHS Executive, Leeds.

19 NHS Confederation (1999) *Spiritual Care in the NHS.* NHS Confederation, Birmingham.

20 National Cancer Alliance (1996) *Patient-Centred Cancer Services? What patients say.* National Cancer Alliance, Oxford.

21 National Council for Hospice and Specialist Palliative Care Services (1995) *Opening Doors: improving access to hospice and specialist palliative care services by members of the black and ethnic minority communities.* Occasional Paper 7. National Council for Hospice and Specialist Palliative Care Services, London.

22 Department of Health (1999) *Compact on Relationships between Government and the Voluntary and Community Sector in England.* HSC 1999/023. DoH, London.

23 NHS Executive (2000) *Manual of Cancer Services Standards.* NHS Executive, Leeds.

24 National Council for Hospice and Specialist Palliative Care Services (1997) *Feeling Better: psychosocial care in specialist palliative care.* Occasional Paper 13. National Council for Hospice and Specialist Palliative Care Services, London.

25 National Council for Hospice and Specialist Palliative Care Services (1998) *Reaching Out: specialist palliative care for adults with non-malignant diseases.* Occasional Paper 14. National Council for Hospice and Specialist Palliative Care Services, London.

26 Thomas K (2000) Out-of-hours palliative care – bridging the gap. *Eur J Palliative Care.* 7: 22–5.

27 Froggatt K (2000) *Palliative Care Education in Nursing Homes, April 2000: an evaluation for Macmillan Cancer Relief and the Registered Nursing Home Association.* Macmillan Cancer Relief, London.

28 National Council for Hospice and Specialist Palliative Care Services (1996) *Education in Palliative Care*. Occasional Paper 9. National Council for Hospice and Specialist Palliative Care Services, London.

29 Barclay SIG, Todd CJ, Grande GE and Lipscombe J (1997) How common is medical training in palliative care? A postal survey of general practitioners. *Br J Gen Pract.* **47**: 800–5.

30 Ward J (2000) *Education requirements in palliative care for GP registrars*. Poster at Royal Society of Medicine Meeting, Scarborough, 5–6 September 2000.

31 Garry AC (1997) The junior doctor's view: a survey to determine influences and concerns for prescribing analgesia in cancer patients. *Palliative Med.* **11**: 79–80. Poster presentation at the Association of Palliative Medicine Conference, Coventry, 6–7 November 1996.

32 Bloxham G, Garry AC and Henderson J (2000) *Psychological, psychiatric and palliation needs of patients within cancer services*. Paper delivered to York Health Services Trust Board, York, 24 July 2000.

33 National Council for Hospice and Specialist Palliative Care Services (1994) *Research in Palliative Care: the pursuit of reliable knowledge*. Occasional Paper 5. National Council for Hospice and Specialist Palliative Care Services, London.

34 National Council for Hospice and Specialist Palliative Care Services (1997) *Making Palliative Care Better: quality improvement, multiprofessional audit and standards*. Occasional Paper 12. National Council for Hospice and Specialist Palliative Care Services, London.

CHAPTER 13

Information, clinical governance and research

Michael Peake and David Forman

Introduction

Every healthcare professional likes to believe that they are doing their best and that they are performing to a high standard. However, where comparative data on performance and outcome for cancer patients in the UK have been available, they have revealed large variations in standards between services. This is the case whether one is comparing the UK with other European countries,[1] one socio-economic group with another within the UK,[2] or making detailed comparisons within a locality.[3] Management gurus tell us that 'information is the key to change'. It is likely that high-quality, clinically relevant information on the performance of one unit in the context of that of regional, national or international peer groups will be more influential in bringing about change than most high-level guidance or edicts. Indeed, the comparative European survival data are widely regarded as a critical driver for the changes in UK cancer services heralded by the Calman–Hine report.[4]

Routine information about cancer in the UK has traditionally come from one of four sources:

1 mortality information from death certifications (the Office for National Statistics in England and Wales and its equivalents in Scotland and Northern Ireland, available since the early part of the twentieth century)
2 incidence and limited treatment information from the regional cancer registries (currently nine in England, together with national registries in each of the other three countries – nationally available since the 1960s)
3 hospital-based discharge information (e.g. Hospital Episode Statistics derived from trust information systems – available since the 1980s)
4 local and certain specialty databases (e.g. for childhood cancers or haematological malignancies and, more recently, for certain common cancers

resulting from clinical initiatives, such as BASO (British Association of Surgical Oncology) for breast cancer and BAHNO (British Association of Head and Neck Oncology) for head and neck cancer). Apart from childhood cancer, this information has not been collected consistently across the country over time.

If we are looking for information to reflect activity, performance and outcome in such a way as to influence practice and the positive development of services, none of the above data sources currently have the scope to meet this requirement. The reasons for this are many, and include the following:

- with some notable exceptions, the lack of case-mix factors makes the comparison of 'like with like' impossible
- the fact that most of the available data are several years old (e.g. in the case of the cancer registries, the most recent information, even in the best regions, can be two years or more out of date), making it easy for trusts and clinicians to discount the results as a legacy of 'old regimes' or discarded sets of practices
- the lack of standardisation of data sets between various units and regions, which adds to the difficulty of making valid inter-unit comparisons
- imperfections in the recording of the cause of death on death certificates
- a lack of clinical confidence in the standard (i.e. the accuracy and completeness) of the data.

The National Performance Indicators published by the NHS Executive are examples of 'high-level' indicators derived from what data are relatively easily available from some of the sources outlined above. There is little doubt that they contain some useful information, but the level of concern about their accuracy, interpretation and lack of timeliness significantly limits their power of influence, and at times they can be positively misleading.

Case-mix factors

In order to be able to compare the healthcare of patients with disease from one area to another, and in particular to assess the standards of referral, diagnosis and treatment between different groupings of clinical services, a knowledge of certain key case-mix variables is essential. Some of the most important variables in the field of cancer include the following:

- age at diagnosis
- sex
- histological type ± grade
- stage at diagnosis
- performance status (i.e. the degree to which symptoms of the disease are restricting activities of daily living)

- comorbidities
- certain other prognostic markers for specific cancer types.

Age and sex are relatively easy data items to collect, but after that it gets difficult. For example, a histological diagnosis is not recorded in about 25% of all cancers,[5] and for some sites (e.g. lung cancer) this figure increases to over 30%. Stage is notoriously under-recorded for many cancers, and even for four 'high-profile' cancers (breast, colorectal, cervix and melanoma) it is only nationally available for half to two-thirds of cancer registrations.[5] Even when present, there is often concern about its accuracy and the classification system utilised. Performance status is one of the most powerful prognostic factors in many cancers, but has to be recorded in 'real time' by an experienced clinician and is very rarely available routinely.

Data sets

The core data sets of the cancer registries across the UK are similar but not the same. For example, some have recorded detailed information about treatment, while others include only minimal information or none at all. This is a result of the historical development of registries as regionally funded and administered bodies with little national co-ordination. Recent initiatives resulting from the NHS Cancer Plan[6] and the NHS Cancer Information Strategy[7] have led to the development of a National Cancer Data Set (NCDS),[8] to be collected by all relevant NHS organisations with regard to their cancer patients. A subset of the NCDS will constitute a new enhanced core data set for the cancer registries.

Several professional groups have also developed, or have been in the process of developing, site-specific clinical data sets for different tumour types,[9–12] while the Royal College of Pathologists has developed a series of site-specific proformas for the systematic reporting of pathological cancer diagnoses.[13] To guard against uncontrolled proliferation of these data sets, and to ensure common standards, over the course of 2001–02 the NCDS Steering Group agreed and published site-specific data sets for all but the rarest cancer types. These incorporate the earlier developments, and the overall intention is to create data sets that serve the needs of clinicians, NHS managers and health organisations as well as those with research interests.

It is vital in any data set that items are clearly *defined* in terms of both their *meaning* and their *purpose*. Awareness of the key *outputs* that are likely to be required from any eventual reporting of the results is an important element in the process of development of the data set. It is intended that collection of this data set will, in time, become mandatory as part of the cancer services accreditation process.

Collecting the data: databases and the like

Agreeing on data sets is the essential starting point for an information system but it is of little value without careful attention to the way in which the data are to be collected. Clinicians record information – usually in writing or by dictation – all the time, but the vast majority of it is unstructured and for most practical purposes is incapable of systematic capture. What is required is nothing short of a *change in the culture* – that is, making routine data collection a normal part of clinical practice. Cancer registry data collectors and research workers may be very experienced in sitting in medical record departments, delving among hospital notes and deciphering doctors' handwriting, but it is hardly the standard that we should be seeking for the future.

Databases that are free-standing and allow only for the retrospective input of data in a rigidly structured format are not the model on which we should be basing systems for the future. Electronic tools need to be developed to be of sufficient use by clinicians to ensure their widespread adoption. With the availability of networked systems in most hospitals, the advances in web technologies and the emergence of cheap, hand-held computers capable of 'wireless' connection to networks, there is no reason why all clinicians should not have access to 'live' databases and clinical management tools, wherever they are working.

Large data sets need to be broken down into sections with regard to when, where and who collects each data item. Care pathways for each cancer site should be examined and those data items which are appropriate to collect at each point on the pathway defined. Such *pathway information nodes* can be further broken down into those which require clinical input and those which do not, thereby further limiting the amount of data that clinicians need to record at any one time. Figure 13.1 shows an example of this in outline for lung cancer.

Additional incentives for clinicians and secretarial staff alike are the generation of useful 'outputs' at each stage of the process. The entry of data items can be used to populate clinic letters, multidisciplinary team meeting reports, referral letters, endoscopy reports, and so on. However, until the production of such outputs becomes a natural part of daily clinical care, their adoption will be restricted to the enthusiasts.

Some of the attributes of an ideal database for these purposes are as follows:

- easy to use – screens designed to mirror routine clinical care as far as possible, and specially designed 'drop-down lists' of options to aid speed, consistency and accuracy
- as much commonality of design as possible between screens for different cancer sites in order to reduce training requirements of clerical and audit staff
- direct links between the databases and the local patient administration systems to avoid the need for double data entry at any level

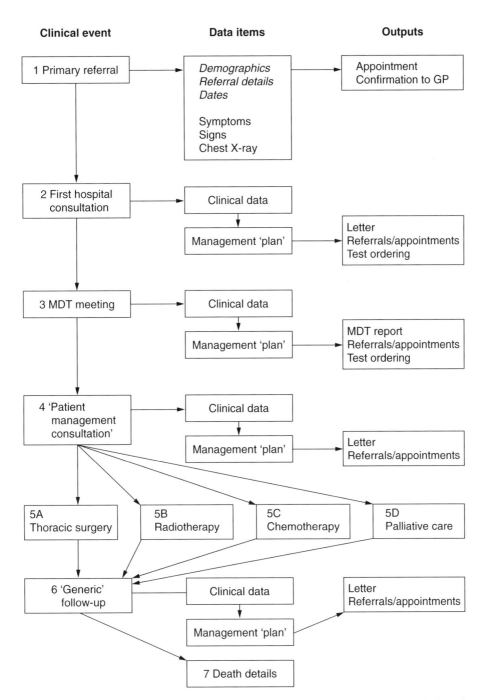

Figure 13.1: Pathway information nodes for lung cancer: summary. MDT = multidisciplinary team.

- well-defined (and common) data-exchange standards to allow the down-loading of data into other systems for the purposes of grouped analysis
- inexpensive enough to allow for near-universal utilisation
- flexible enough to allow for the local development of new screens and data items without corrupting the 'core' database, and without the need to employ professional programmers
- Web enabled
- meeting or exceeding NHS standards of security and confidentiality
- including tools to aid control of the quality of the data
- containing built-in access to 'help texts' and other supportive material to act as real-time educational tools
- options for free-text comments with regard to specific unusual patient or tumour characteristics.

Electronic patient records

It is NHS policy to work towards an electronic patient record (EPR) over the next few years, and such a development should have the capability to contribute greatly to the aims outlined above. However, it will continue to be important to keep in mind the different functions of core data sets for comparative audit, clinical management systems and a comprehensive EPR. Such all-embracing electronic records are very likely to become as difficult to probe and as open to interpretation as traditional written records if we ignore the need for careful structuring of the information within them.

Collating, analysing and reporting of grouped data

The numbers of patients who are managed by an individual clinician or even a clinical unit over a period of time that is short enough to allow for timely feed-back are likely to be too small to be of much value for assessing reliably any of the more important outcomes, if analysed in isolation. One of the great strengths of larger groupings of data is not only the comparisons that can be made, but also the statistical power that is associated with larger numbers. There will, of course, be important local issues (e.g. audits of performance against agreed standards) that are well suited to analysis at the unit level, at least in the first instance. However, it is clear that cancer *networks* are becoming increasingly important, especially since the intention is for common protocols and guidelines to be implemented across the cancer centres and units within each network.

This makes the network the natural first level of collation above the unit or centre. Above this there will be the need for *regional* comparisons and finally *national* and *international* comparisons will complete the picture.

The cancer registries have until now been the only bodies with a systematic brief in this area, and their place within this evolving process needs to be carefully worked out. Their great strength has been in defining the population 'denominator' of a particular cancer type, without which proper comparisons of outcomes are impossible. The debate surrounding the validity of comparative survival analyses across Europe[7] is to a large extent based on the degree to which the outcomes from each country can be said to be truly representative of those of the population in general.

Whatever information systems are developed within the NHS in the short term, it will be the registries (in collaboration with the Office for National Statistics and equivalent organisations in Scotland and Northern Ireland) that have to provide the population-based 'context' for the resulting reports. Registries will have to adapt to meet the new demands placed upon them by expanded data sets, and such a development has been described in a new Action Programme for Cancer Registries.[14] This emphasises the importance of registries capturing electronically the relevant components of the NCDS, and shifting their resources away from data acquisition and warehousing and towards quality assurance and added-value analysis and research.

In this context, it is worth stating that such population-based research can only succeed if the data that are analysed are truly population based. One potential major threat to this sine qua non is the requirement for the process of cancer registration to be based on explicit patient-informed consent. Although superficially attractive, the inherent problems in such a universal consent process would fatally undermine the population basis of the data.[15] Cancer is diagnosed in a wide variety of different environments, often in stressful circumstances, and not all of these would lend themselves to obtaining consent routinely. There is no population-based cancer registration system in the world that successfully operates using informed consent. Complete and unbiased coverage of the entire population would be lost if consent were made mandatory.

Professional ownership and clinical governance

If such a programme of data collection and analysis becomes an entirely management-led initiative without clinical input, it is likely to fail on many important levels. Clinicians will only be supportive – or indeed enthusiastic – if they respect the nature and quality of what is collected and the individuals who are analysing and interpreting the results. This begs the question of 'Who is the information for?'. Clearly, it is ultimately for the benefit of patients. If this process does not lead to improved standards of care, it will have been a waste of effort.

Clinical governance is all about improving clinical standards in an open, information-rich environment. It has been described as 'the corporate accountability for clinical performance'.[16] Clinicians in general welcome the principles underlying the concept, but the problem is that in the past they have had little reason to be confident about the standard of the information upon which such judgements might be made. It is therefore in their interests to support high-quality data collection and analysis. The need for *professional ownership* of the process is not therefore a form of protectionism, but simply the recognition that the issues are complex and require great knowledge and experience within a particular field if sense is to be made of information of this nature.

Access to reports

It is clear that properly measured and analysed performance and outcome indicators should be freely available to the purchasers and consumers of healthcare. Whether such information, at this stage in the development of the data collection business, should access the performance of individual doctors rather than *clinical teams* seems less clear. The emergence of the properly structured multidisciplinary team has been one of the major successes of the Calman–Hine initiative, and should probably be the lowest level to which information on performance is published for general consumption. However, there may be occasions when analysis of the performance of individual practitioners will be appropriate as part of legitimate audit and quality assurance mechanisms.

The publishing of league tables is fraught with problems unless they are properly interpreted. There is already evidence of cardiac surgical units refusing to operate on higher-risk patients for fear of harming their published mortality rates. Such a trend has to be counter-productive in the long term, especially in the context of an ageing population where there is already evidence of ageism in cancer treatments.[17,18]

Data collection and research

Assuming that this idealised data-rich environment does become a reality, then in theory it will be possible to measure the effects of many interventions in ways that would only have been possible by detailed and limited research protocols in the past. One model is the field of haemato-oncology, where such a high percentage of patients with leukaemia and lymphoma in the UK have been entered into national multicentre trials that it could be argued, for practical purposes, such a situation already exists.

It has been assumed that research – and in this context we are referring mainly to the phase III clinical trial – is the ultimate way of establishing the evidence on which to base clinical practice. However, such trials only examine limited therapeutic issues and groups of patients. Entry to trials is limited by strict inclusion and exclusion criteria, and only includes patients who consent to take part. Such patients are often not fully representative of those who are seen in wider clinical practice. In addition, only such investigations and other variables that are predetermined to be of importance in the design phase of the study are recorded, potentially further limiting the general applicability of the results. The measurement of outcomes of therapeutic interventions in large populations where good case-mix variables and the population 'denominator' are known could, at least in theory, provide critical complementary evidence alongside phase III trials.

Summary

The routine collection of carefully selected data items together with their collation, analysis and timely reporting at network, regional, national and international levels should be a powerful force for improving the standards of cancer and other clinical services in the UK. Such ongoing comparative audit will contribute greatly to clinical governance. Such a process needs to be clinically 'owned' but open and accountable to commissioners of healthcare, the NHS Executive and patients. The contribution of the cancer registries is crucial in obtaining a population-based perspective on such information, and their role in such a process in the future needs careful consideration. The analogies between phase III clinical trials and this process, together with their relative strengths and weaknesses, is a topic worthy of further debate.

References

1 Berrino F, Capocaccia J, Estève J *et al.* (1999) *Survival of Cancer Patients in Europe: the Eurocare-2 Study.* IARC Scientific Publications No 151. International Agency for Research on Cancer, Lyon.

2 Coleman MP, Babb P, Damiecki P *et al.* (2000) *Cancer Survival Trends.* Office for National Statistics, London.

3 Northern and Yorkshire Cancer Registration and Information Service (1998–2000) *Cancer Treatment Policies and Their Effects on Survival: key sites studies, 1998–2000.* NYCRIS, Leeds.

4 http://www.doh.gov.uk/cancer/calmanhine.htm

5 UK Association of Cancer Registries (2000) *Quality and Performance Indicators.* Unpublished report. Cancer Unit, Office for National Statistics, London.

6 http://www.doh.gov.uk/cancer/cancerplan.htm

7 http://www.doh.gov.uk/cancer/cis.htm

8 http://www.cancer.nhsia.nhs.uk/dataset/

9 http://www.cancernw.org.uk/clinit/products_baso.htm

10 Royal College of Physicians (1999) *Lung Cancer: a core data set.* Royal College of Physicians, London.

11 http://www.cancernw.org.uk/clinit/products_acp.htm

12 British Association of Head and Neck Oncologists (1999) *National Minimum and Advisory Head and Neck Cancer Data Sets.* British Association of Head and Neck Oncologists, London.

13 http://www.rcpath.org/activities/list.html

14 http://www.doh.gov.uk/cancer/actionprogramme.htm

15 Brewster DH, Coleman MP, Forman D and Roche M (2000) Cancer information under threat: the case for legislation. *Ann Oncol.* **12**: 145–7.

16 Watkins P (1999) Clinical governance. *J R Coll Phys Lond.* **33**: 201.

17 Thompson S, Lowe D, Pearson MG and Peake MD (2000) Impact of age on treatment and survival in lung cancer. *Am J Resp Crit Care Med.* **161**: A766.

18 Peake MD, Cartman ML, Muers MF and Forman D (2000) Management of lung cancer in the elderly. *Am J Resp Crit Care Med.* **161**: A766.

CHAPTER 14

The future of cancer services: aspirations for the cancer patient

Mark R Baker

Introduction

The foregoing chapters have described the changes which are required in services in order to implement the benefits that are aspired to in the Calman–Hine Report and subsequent national guidance. These changes will reshape many aspects of hospital and community health services in the interests of patients with cancer, and the associated improvements in the process of care are expected to lead to improvements in both survival and quality of life. Although these are laudable objectives in themselves, and are clearly important to patients and their families, survival is not everything. The lives of many patients with cancer are blighted not only by their disease but also by their experiences during the process of diagnosis and treatment. Improving the process of care for cancer patients and their families is a legitimate goal in its own right, and is not necessarily dependent on a demonstrable impact on survival.

The inability of the NHS to grow as fast as demand has resulted in the experience of most patients being dominated by waiting. Excess of demand over supply and inefficiencies in delivering care are not unique to the NHS, but their combination and extent result in waiting being the cardinal characteristic of public sector healthcare in the UK. Eliminating unnecessary waiting, substantially reducing the duration of each phase of the process of diagnosis and treatment, and guaranteeing access to specialist care when it is required are such obvious requirements that they have been taken for granted and not actually delivered. Massive improvements in these areas are now required, and they will have a significant impact on patients' experience of healthcare, although expectations are still so low that they are too easily met. As patients' experience of services overseas increases, their expectations of healthcare in this country will grow and put further pressure on NHS resources and targets.

Of comparable importance, but less easily measured, is the style of care offered to patients. Here there is less evidence that the UK's experience is significantly worse than that overseas, although this may be due to universal failure in this area rather than to a relatively better performance by the NHS. The Government's approach to dealing with the quality of the process of care is driven by a belief in the empowerment of patients, encouraging greater involvement in their individual care and decisions about their care. A good way of looking at this is for the clinicians and managers who are involved in the delivery and organisation of cancer services to ask themselves 'Would we be satisfied with this care ourselves or for members of our families?' Too often the answer to that question is no, and too rarely is anything done about it. Intolerance of professional arrogance and poor communication is starting to take root in our society and is never likely to lessen. It is imperative that services respond with openness and sensitivity if patient dissatisfaction, which turns into distress, is to be reduced.

Surviving well

In simple terms, the objective of the changes that are now being introduced in cancer care is to increase survival by about 10%. Overall, cancer patients in the UK have a 36% chance of surviving five years, compared with 46% in the top quartile of European countries. By increasing specialist care and investing in cancer services capacity, it is hoped that this gap can be narrowed and eventually eliminated by midway through the next decade. It is less easy to measure improvements in the quality of survival and to ensure that better cancer results are due to a prolongation of life rather than a prolongation of death. The close and early involvement of palliative care specialists for all or almost all cancer patients is important not just for the management of terminal care, but for dealing with the many physical and psychological traumas which cancer patients experience, whether or not their cancer kills them.

All change

At every level, from the patient–clinician relationship to strategic organisations, role changes are occurring with ever-increasing frequency. I shall now outline some of the new roles expected of organisations and individuals involved in cancer services.

Strategic health authorities

Strategic health authorities were established in April 2002 to replace two tiers of management at the intermediate level between the operational NHS and the Department of Health. In many respects, strategic health authorities are the new regions covering populations of 1.5 to 2.5 million and exercising the responsibilities previously invested in regional offices of the NHS Executive. Their role in cancer services is primarily to handle the performance management of those organisations that are responsible for the commissioning and delivery of cancer services (NHS trusts and primary care trusts). They will also have responsibilities for the development of clinical networks, including cancer networks, and could well become the hosts for these organisations. Strategic health authorities are important organisations but, as they do not have control of either finance or staffing, they may well find that they lack the leverage to exercise their responsibilities effectively.

Cancer networks

As described elsewhere, cancer networks are charged with the responsibility for implementing the NHS Cancer Plan. Referred to in passing in the Calman–Hine Report, and adopted subsequently as the standard terminology for joint working for hospitals in Scotland, clinical networks have become the Holy Grail of service improvement throughout the UK. However, devoid of a detailed definition networks are whatever observers want them to be, with ill-defined roles and purpose and confused accountability. Yet in the field of cancer their structure and accountability are defined in sufficient detail in the *Manual of Cancer Services Standards*, and their responsibilities are detailed in the NHS Cancer Plan. The problems that they face are rather more subtle than this.

As non-statutory organisations, they can best be regarded as member organisations, the members being those commissioners and providers of cancer care within their area. By having responsibility for implementing the NHS Cancer Plan, including the full implementation of *Improving Outcomes Guidance*, they face potential conflict with the parochial interests of their own members. Resolving paradoxes like this while keeping all of the members on board requires a level of political leadership which few networks can call upon. Only by aligning themselves with strategic health authorities can the paradox be resolved, but then cancer networks will be caught between the performance management responsibilities of strategic health authorities and the service development responsibilities of their members and themselves.

Cancer units

Most district general hospitals are designated as cancer units and, having achieved that status around 1997, expected to be left alone to get on with their work. In practice, the full implementation of recent *Improving Outcomes Guidance* and the revisiting of the guidance on common cancers calls these assumptions into question. Indeed, the future role and scope of district general hospitals are under serious review, largely as a result of the changes in cancer care. Until the late 1990s, the move had been systematically to encourage local general hospitals to deliver as wide a range of services as possible, and to encourage individual clinicians to innovate and develop new services. In recent years and for the foreseeable future this process is going into reverse, with the elimination of uncontrolled innovation, the consolidation and centralisation of low-frequency and high-skill services, and an overall reduction in the scope of district general hospitals. Needless to say, these trends have not been universally well received. Although the pessimists have overestimated the impact of these trends on the viability of general hospitals, there is no doubt that the role and functions of district general hospitals will have to be revised downwards. What is important for patients is that district general hospitals do the basics well, and that they refer on appropriately to hospitals where additional expertise is available for those who require it.

The recent consolidation of NHS trust structures following the merger of hospital trusts has created a number of organisations which are large in their own right, offering hospital services for populations of half a million or more. These new and large organisations understandably believe that they will be able to offer a wider range of services than their predecessors. In practice, many of these aspirations will be dashed. Serving the interests of patients means that district general hospitals must aspire to excellence in the range of services which it is appropriate for them to provide, and not seek to expand in areas where their workload will never be sufficient to enable them to offer services of very high added value. The competitiveness of the NHS internal market and the personal aspirations of the managers and clinicians in local trusts will not easily be relegated, and longstanding tension can be anticipated between the aspirations of units and the roles assigned to them by policy makers.

Cancer centres

The concept behind the role and definition of a cancer centre among the authors of the Calman–Hine Report was a specialist centre serving a population of two million or more. This idea had to be diluted somewhat in order to secure the signature of the Welsh representatives on the Committee, leading to a halving of the population size. In practice, some cancer centres serve populations even smaller than this, and in practice offer little more than cancer-unit facilities with radiotherapy. This rather defeats the object.

During the accreditation process for cancer centres, which was conducted in the late 1990s, it became clear that few if any aspiring cancer centres offered the facilities and skills envisaged in the Calman–Hine Report, and that substantial development was required throughout the country to enable the capacity, specialisation and expertise to be developed. With the emergence of cancer networks as managed organisations, cancer centres should now be seen as part of the network rather than as the hub of it. They have a role which is greater than that of a cancer unit, but they do not have a controlling interest over the whole network. In addition, of course, cancer centres almost invariably carry out the responsibilities of cancer units for their local population. It is frequently observed that the demands of establishing the cancer centre functions have distracted attention from developing cancer unit services and facilities. It is interesting to note that many cancer centres regard their network as excessively focused on the needs of cancer units, whereas almost invariably cancer units regard their network as centre focused. Perhaps this implies that the balance of power and influence is just about right.

Primary care trusts

Primary care trusts were originally created in order to manage primary care. Subsequent revolution in the organisation of the health service means that, from April 2002, primary care trusts in England will effectively become the new health authorities. They will have comprehensive responsibilities for commissioning specialist services and for providing primary and community care services. They will be the principal focus for public health action, working closely with local authorities, and they will receive financial allocations direct from the Department of Health. They are, incidentally, too small and ill equipped to perform any of these functions effectively. Notwithstanding their history and early difficulties, primary care trusts are the future, and the model provides an appropriate basis for developing local health services. They do need to 'size up' and 'skill up' during the next year or two in order to be able to fulfil their functions, but they are essentially a good idea.

Primary care trusts will have clinical cancer leads, like cancer units, centres and networks, and they will have responsibilities for improving the role of primary care in cancer pathways, as well as for informing the commissioning and development of services in hospitals. It is essential that primary care trusts are full members of cancer networks and that their clinical leads are afforded the same status and opportunities as lead clinicians in cancer units.

The intrinsic risk is that primary care trusts will be entirely focused on the needs of their local units and oblivious to the roles and aspirations of the local cancer centre. They could therefore become another set of obstacles to implementing service reconfiguration and to getting the centres right. Hence the importance of involving primary care trust cancer leads as fully and effectively as possible in the work of the cancer network as a whole, and ensuring that they are fully briefed and sharing ownership of specialist service planning and commissioning.

The cancer patient

Patients with cancer and their carers should not be passive recipients of all the change described above. At the heart of modernisation is the empowerment of the customer/user, and cancer patients are – first and foremost – users of services. The hopes and fears, aspirations and expectations of patients need to be central to decisions about their care and where they might receive it. Contrary to the claims of those in local hospitals who seek to maintain the status quo, people with serious illness are often prepared to travel long distances in discomfort in order to obtain the best possible quality of care. When the reasons for reconfiguring services are fully explained, patients are usually supportive so long as they have confidence that services will improve as a result.

Too little attention has been paid to developing information for patients about their disease in general and their own care in particular. The development and use of patient-held records and the systematic presentation of information about their disease and the treatment pathways is an important means of empowering patients in the professional–client relationship. The reluctance of many clinicians to use these vehicles and the customary refusal of doctors to write in patient-held records is as much to do with power as to do with time. These problems will not be overcome quickly or easily, but they will eventually be overcome. Patient empowerment is here to stay – it is important and valuable, it is the right thing to do, and it will improve compliance with and completion of care programmes. In any case, for patients to be consulted about their care and for them to make informed decisions about their care is a right, not a privilege.

Clinicians

The role of the clinician in cancer care is changing, too. In nursing and medicine, in radiography and medical physics, in psychology and the therapies and in non-surgical oncology, subject and site specialisation have become mandatory and specialist training programmes have narrowed. All are now expected to work in teams, and time has to be allocated within the working week for multidisciplinary team meetings and mandatory audit and clinical governance processes. Patients' expectations and the time allowed for consultations are increasing, and the need to communicate effectively has become paramount. Departures from protocol-based care have to be explained and justified, and service innovation has to be officially authorised. Life will never be quite the same again.

The step from senior specialist registrar to consultant has always been a giant leap, but with reductions in the period of training the step is greater than ever. Many new consultants, especially those working in subspecialised fields, will require a period of supervision by a senior colleague, and will continue to learn aspects of decision making as well as technical skills for many years. Their more senior colleagues will have greater experience, but may not be used to the narrowness of the new jobs required. While specialists in the past have enjoyed an evolving role, the opportunities may now be limited by the difficulty in replacing them in their specialist field, and the non-transferability of much of their experience.

The external pressures on professional staff engendered by clinical governance and the mounting exposure of service failures increase the pressure on all concerned and heighten the issue of clinical accountability. In these circumstances, a much greater commitment to continuing professional education and peer support is necessary to maintain and develop the quality of care and to ensure that staff are attracted to these posts.

Conclusion

From the cancer patient's point of view, the changes now being introduced into the NHS are long overdue and much to be welcomed. What is surprising, perhaps, is that it has taken so long for the deficiencies in cancer care in the UK to become apparent and for concerted action to redress them to be introduced.

From the standpoint of those responsible for managing and delivering care, this is not a matter of apportioning blame but rather of ensuring that the future is immeasurably better than the past. What must be absolutely clear in everybody's mind is that the opportunities presented by the National Cancer Strategy constitute an opportunity that cannot and must not be missed.

Index